Praise for *No Such Thing as Normal*

'Bigg meticulously documents how pervasive and harmful psychiatry's biomedical vision continues to be, while guiding us toward more compassionate responses to human suffering' **Professor Justin Garson, author of** *Madness* **and** *The Madness Pill*

'Written with sharp insight and unflinching clarity, this book is more than a critique – it is a call to action for a more honest and compassionate response to mental distress, one that is both possible and urgently needed' **Dr Samara Linton, co-editor of** *The Colour of Madness*

'A really much-needed contribution' **Nick Dearden, author of** *Pharmanomics*

'This book made me revaluate everything I thought I knew about psychiatric care, challenging some of the most fundamental assumptions about mental health, and showing how a radically new approach to "normality" is needed' **Emma Szewczak, author of** *The Stich Up*

'Amazingly well done and an insightful read – a must-have if you want to look past what is defined as "normal"' **Dr Nighat Arif, author of** *The Knowledge*

'A rallying cry for an approach to mental health that is informed by the circumstances, experiences and diversity of those of us who struggle. I have never read a clearer case for the importance of social and systemic approaches to psychiatric distress' **Emma Byrne, author of** *Swearing is Good for You*

NO SUCH THING AS NORMAL

Disorders, Diagnoses
and the Limits of Psychiatry

MARIEKE BIGG

Profile Books

First published in Great Britain in 2025 by
Profile Books Ltd
29 Cloth Fair
London
ECIA 7JQ
www.profilebooks.com

Copyright © Marieke Bigg, 2025

1 3 5 7 9 10 8 6 4 2

Typeset in Berling Nova Text by MacGuru Ltd
Printed and bound in Great Britain by
CPI Group (UK) Ltd, Croydon CRO 4YY

A CIP catalogue record for this book is available from the British Library.

We make every effort to make sure our products are safe for the purpose
for which they are intended. For more information check our website
or contact Authorised Rep Compliance Ltd., Ground Floor, 71 Lower
Baggot Street, Dublin, D02 P593, Ireland, www.arccompliance.com

ISBN 978 1 80081 901 6
eISBN 978 1 80081 905 4

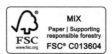

To the parts of ourselves we learn to love.

Contents

Introduction

Psychiatry and Society: A Mental Health Tragedy

Most of us today have either had our own experience with, or know someone with, a mental health problem. More so than any other time, mental health is a topic on our tongues and on our minds. There is talk of a crisis. Opinions are divided about whether mental disorder is actually on the rise.[1] Whatever your view, around a billion people are living with a mental, neurological or substance-use disorder today.[2] People are diagnosed more than ever before; once psychiatric disease was a marginal matter, today it affects us all.

The crisis is often discussed in epidemiological terms, as a population problem, not an individual problem. People explain the rising rates by pointing to pandemics, social isolation and austerity. They talk about mental disease, or disorder, as linked to the world that causes us to suffer.

We intuitively understand that people don't suffer in a vacuum. That things happen to people to make them feel a certain way. And yet, somehow, we continue to think about the appropriate solutions for mental distress in individual medical terms. Rather than turning to the structural problems that we have all seen as somehow connected with the state of our minds, we continue to think of mental health as personal responsibility. We are told to care for our minds the way we care for our bodies.

We are told to see a doctor, get a prescription, and find a way to cope.

At the heart of the medical view of mental suffering is the field of psychiatry. Spokespeople for psychiatry have made some bold promises over the past decades, to cure mental illness with its medical solutions. Despite the scientific breakthroughs reported in the media, about genes found, brain patterns identified, or new cutting-edge drugs, these don't seem to be making much of a difference to the amassing new cases.[3] As much as the field has undoubtedly offered a lifeline to many, there are so many others it hasn't helped, and there is no way that we could possibly claim to have eradicated mental suffering with drugs or other medical technology. If its aim has been to cure mental disorder, psychiatry hasn't exactly achieved its objective. And yet we keep turning to its methods.

All this stems from an inconvenient truth at the foundation of our understanding of mental health: the mental disorders we today make sense of as illnesses akin to diabetes or arthritis still have no proven biological cause. There is no catch-all explanation rooted in genetics or the brain for any of the psychiatric diseases that have been defined by modern psychiatry. While we can use drugs to mitigate symptoms, it is doubtful that we will ever use them to cure psychosis or depression in any straightforward way.

There *is*, on the other hand, a proven link between the world we live in and the state of our minds. And yet, this view is often discredited by the profession with the means and influence to push for social changes that will help.

Both the United Nations (UN) and the World Health Organisation (WHO) have now recognised that the bio-medical model for mental health is falling short and, importantly, that the social determinants of mental health need urgent attention.[4] WHO have even called for a total overhaul of the medical model in mental health.[5] This medical model in its current form isn't meeting the needs of people who are suffering mentally across the globe. And yet we continue to prescribe drugs and treat mental distress as exclusively biological conditions. Antidepressant drug prescriptions are only on the rise.[6] Psychiatric drug sales overall have increased internationally, at an average of 4 per cent annually between 2008 and 2019.[7]

Psychiatry is failing us, yet it is a growing, steadily powerful force shaping our economy, our society, and our very sense of self.

With numerous pronouncements in recent years, even from within the psychiatric community itself, that the discipline is based on a discredited and defunct set of beliefs, it is surprising that money and demand continue to flow. The profession has achieved what some psychiatrists have called a 'cult-like' status, in that it has insisted on untruths, has found ways to exercise control over psychiatrist-dissenters who have spoken out or pulled away, and continues to proselytise aggressively against the tide of scientific findings that contradict its approach. All this, while also manipulating its messaging to the outside world through the mechanisms of a powerful authority vested in a bible under the title of the Diagnostic and Statistical Manual of Mental Disorders (DSM), published by the American Psychiatric Association.[8] While this bunker-like mentality was noted as far back as sixty years ago,[9] the profession has clung to its methods, and has continued to find financial and political support, far beyond what is justifiable in terms of human benefit.

By delineating a narrow field of vision in which it could claim sole authority, psychiatry has grown in influence and scope. Endorsed by governments, it has shaped public understanding of mental disease as individual and biologically rooted, garnering support while detracting from the conditions that we know perpetuate mental distress, and entrench inequality.

Because as well as an inconvenient truth, there is also an injustice at the heart of the mental health crisis: it is worse among groups of people who are marginalised or discriminated against. This has a lot to do with the conditions they live in. Women in the UK are 10 times as likely as men to have experienced extensive physical and sexual abuse during their lives; in the US, 9 out of 10 victims of rape are female.[10] UK statistics show that 26 per cent of victims of sexual abuse have tried to take their life, and 22 per cent have self-harmed.[11] Research from across the world shows that these predominantly female victims are very likely to experience post-traumatic stress disorder, or suicidal ideation, as well as other mental health conditions like schizophrenia or depression as a result of their abuse.[12] This likelihood increases for women of colour. When women do find themselves diagnosed, mental health support is generally lacking. In the UK, only 1 in 3 people who experience mental health problems are able to access the support they need[13]; in the US, the figure is as high as 4 in 10,[14] yet groups facing particularly high levels of poor mental health – those who are also already disadvantaged in other aspects of their lives – also often experience the greatest difficulty in accessing services. In both the UK and the US, minoritised groups are the least likely to access the help they need – whether medication for mental health, counselling or therapy.[15]

Looking at gender disparities in mental health in particular brings the inequality in mental health into high relief. Globally, women and girls are nearly twice as likely as boys and men to suffer from mental ill health.[16] This disparity is echoed, to a greater or lesser degree, across almost every mental condition. UK and US studies show that women are twice as likely to be diagnosed with anxiety or depression as men. Women are 3 times as likely to be diagnosed with an eating disorder. 25.7 per cent of women as opposed to 9.7 per cent of men aged 16 to 24 report having self-harmed at some point in their life.[17] In the cases where women are diagnosed less often, this doesn't mean they aren't suffering, only often that they are underdiagnosed because male criteria are being applied with no regard for how these might manifest differently in women. US research suggests that men are 4 times more likely than women to be diagnosed with autism.[18] Some research suggests that as many as 80 per cent of autistic women are missed.[19] Often, they are initially misdiagnosed with more 'typically female' conditions like anxiety disorders, depression and mood disorders, borderline personality disorder, obsessive compulsive disorder and eating disorders.

Other disorders still, like post-traumatic stress disorder, that have always been studied and understood with a male patient in mind, are now increasingly being diagnosed in women, but with little understanding of the specific social conditions in which they arise. These are conditions that exist outside of psychiatry's gendered caricatures, like ghosts haunting them with the limitations of the profession.

And yet, psychiatry continues to thrive.

Where there is contradiction there is often power holding incommensurate opposites in place. When we zoom out on the state of psychiatry, those power dynamics become clear. We see why, in the context of global capitalism, a profession vested in marketable solutions was preferable over social changes that would compromise the profits of the wealthy few.

In the context of a history of patriarchy, colonialism and other forms of oppression, too, we see how countless minds of the already disenfranchised could be easily sacrificed to maintaining the status quo. Psychiatry has long provided an authoritative explanation for people's suffering that has nothing to do with the system that fails them, and placed the deficiency in the bodies of implicitly inferior individuals. In doing so, it has isolated us with our suffering, and exacerbated the self-blame and shame that conveniently prevents us from sharing, and so possibly exposing the systematic scope of our distress.

It seems absurd to think that a mind can exist independently, in complete disconnect from the physical world around it, but that is what modern psychiatry makes us believe. To rectify the problem of our sad, stressed and isolated minds we need to reconfigure our image of mental disorder, to put it back in the world, and to bring to light the problem where it truly lives. We may not be facing a mental health crisis after all, but a crisis in our social and mental healthcare systems that needs an urgent remedy.

In this book I want to chart the cost that we pay to uphold a solely psychiatric, medicalised view of mental distress and experience. I want to show who suffers as a result of this view's shortcomings, how they suffer, and what it would take for psychiatry to help.

We will explore how psychiatry diagnoses and treats human experience, and how psychiatric thinking has created a system that prioritises policing gendered and racial stereotypes over answering the questions that would help its patients the most. We see how this has allowed some of psychiatry's nineteenth-century, most pejorative constructs to survive. Take hysteria, which, in its modern guises, is often used to discredit the impact of the traumas women face by placing the cause and deficiency in their bodies and minds, rather than the violence they experience. This stands in contrast to the story of post-traumatic stress disorder (PTSD) that validates the violence experienced by men in warfare.

Many of psychiatry's faulty concepts have survived due to financial backing. In modern times, financial imperative helps explain how a pharmaceutical industry and extensive government marketing efforts have secured a narrow, brain-based, biochemical view of mental suffering that may not be offering us the answers we need.

Financial imperative, political incentive and historic prejudice combine to shape many of the common understandings in psychiatry today. Borderline personality disorder (BPD) is one of psychiatry's most contested diagnoses. BPD today is diagnosed predominantly in women deemed angry or resistant to treatment. We'll unpick how prejudice has trumped science with these labels, and what it would take to instead help people to cope with the traumatising realities of their lives.

Biological psychiatry does not tell the full story of mental distress. We follow one of the most gendered diagnoses, postpartum depression (PPD), to show that it isn't as exclusive to women as the DSM makes us think and masks the inordinate social expectations placed on mothers. The side effects of all these conditions are not only social disadvantage in material terms, but also internalised stigma and shame that undermine the sense of agency that is so essential to healing. Cases like PPD point to places where cultural assumptions, rather than human benefit, can easily drive research and care when psychiatrists cling too tightly to the power and legitimacy vested in their biological approach. This leads those working in the field to miss opportunities to help that might fall outside their purview. We'll see this in the most explicit form in the case of psychopathy; especially female psychopathy, which has reinforced ideas about inherent biological difference that is of little help to the individuals and their families. Psychopathy shows us the extreme consequences of asserting an uninterrogated biological view; here asserting and reinforcing social power structures through incarceration, precluding the possibility of rehabilitation, choosing instead to control.

We'll open up to a broader perspective, drawing on the case of schizophrenia, and begin to expose the social determinants of mental distress, especially among minoritised groups, and how medical diagnoses obscure the need for social reform, as well as more humane and more helpful forms of support. We'll also look to psychedelics, long seen as a countercultural alternative to pharmaceuticals, that today are being embraced by mainstream psychiatry. There is an opportunity, here, to learn from these previously marginalised practices, and use them to meet the needs of people who have also been sidelined. There is a risk, though, that financial incentive, once again, will pave the way. This likelihood is evident in the ways that these alternatives to western medicine have been periodically invented, rejected, and now greedily embraced by an industry wary of losing control of its medically sanctioned, highly profitable sector. We explore what it would mean to learn from excluded perspectives. We'll turn to autism, too, now more often diagnosed in women than it has previously been (though still highly under-diagnosed), to ask what we can learn from autistic people about adequate support. The research currently focused on deficits, the ways in which autistic people fall short of a norm, for example, may not be the most pressing. Perhaps research on how they process and experience the world will be more interesting. Maybe we need to augment treatment currently emphasising the behavioural adjustment of people with autism, with social changes to better facilitate a range of cognitive processing styles. When we listen to these voices, we find that the goals of psychiatric research shift; that they might be less about 'curing' difference, and more about supporting individuals with their unique and equally valid experience.

This leads us to a vision of a different psychiatry; of psychiatry embedded in a mental healthcare system rather than reigning over it. This system is premised on connection over oppression, on supportive relationships over prescriptions, on people's experiences over diagnoses, on collaboration between services over fragmentation. We imagine a profession that, rather than conspiring with a social order that atomises, takes responsibility for social neglect, and offers a systemic, individualised approach to supporting people to live meaningful and connected lives. And in doing so, psychiatry, too, could become a powerful engine for social change.

Mental health crisis or not, mental illnesses are specific inflections of human suffering. Neuroscientific research continues to confirm what Freud already knew – that we all have the propensity for madness. Given the right triggers – a sufficiently hostile environment – we can all slide along that slippery spectrum of human coping strategies in an attempt to meet the challenges of our lives. And so it makes sense that these coping strategies will differ depending on the environment in which we find ourselves, and it makes sense that those who find themselves in a particularly hostile environment will likely need to adapt more starkly. We need to understand how the world shapes minds, to treat mental distress as a social disease. We also need to understand how individuals can work with the world to heal their minds from distress, and we need to understand how we can shape the world to alleviate mental suffering.

Above all, what drives recovery is the taste of something better. This book is about the madness that connects us, and how, in a world that creates the conditions of our experience, we can find answers that might lead to personal and social change.

1

Hysteria, PTSD and the Birth of Psychiatry

While hysteria has existed through the ages, it wasn't always a psychiatric diagnosis. It began as a gynaecological disease, with early uses of the term in ancient Egypt referring to the havoc wreaked by a wandering womb, causing women to behave erratically. Over time, modifications of this gynaecological explanation were used to explain other gender-defying symptoms, like a refusal to have children or marry. Hysteria emerged again in the late nineteenth century, this time as a neurological disease. The symptoms of hysteria, by this point, were well known: emotional lability, mental fits, paralysis, loss of sensation and convulsions, an affliction that seemed to affect predominantly White, affluent women, and had a sexual overtone. And the symptoms look fairly similar in the modern psychiatric manuals of mental disorders. The Diagnostic and Statistical Manual of Mental Disorders (DSM), the psychiatric manual used largely in the US to guide clinicians with diagnosis, still lists symptoms that closely resemble those long associated with hysteria under a new term, histrionic personality disorder (HPD). A person with HPD might present with attention-seeking and seductive behaviour, emotional instability, a dramatic way of expression and emotional neediness.[1]

While hysteria has existed as a female disease from the

earliest days of western civilisation, the roots for modern-day hysteria were really consolidated in the nineteenth century. At a time when psychiatry was still nascent, psychiatrists sought to assert their profession as on par with medicine. In the era of Enlightenment science, an era of objective truths and empirical evidence, this meant finding a biological basis to classified conditions in the same way medicine had.

One doctor in particular, Jean-Martin Charcot, who took up his post as the chair of pathology at the Salpêtrière hospital in 1872, laid the groundwork for systematic investigations into the root of the disease. He didn't consider hysteria to be a gynaecological disease like many of his colleagues and predecessors; he and his followers were convinced that the cause was located in the brain. Charcot was a neurologist, which meant that he had a very particular method. He called his approach 'clinico-anatomic': he would deduce patterns of symptoms across various patients, and once those patients died, he would dissect their brains. These dissections would, in theory, show associations or commonalities between patients presenting the same symptoms, potentially offering insight into the cause of the disease itself. If he could connect the symptom to a common physical abnormality, he would have a generalisable scheme for diagnosis.

This approach had proved successful for Charcot in deducing many neurological conditions, not least multiple sclerosis. But when he turned his attention to hysteria, it didn't yield the results he expected. He wanted to understand this disorder. He wanted to investigate, given its symptomatic similarity to the epilepsy of patients who coinhabited the hospital, whether this was a discrete condition from epilepsy. And he was convinced that this was a biological, physical condition with a root that could be found in the brains of the patients he diagnosed.

As it turned out, the post-mortem brains of hysterical patients were structurally completely normal.[2]

Not to be dissuaded, Charcot doubled down. He believed that better microscopes and new techniques would eventually reveal the defects of hysterical brains; it was just a matter of time and technology. In the meantime, he focused his efforts on the patients' presenting symptoms, which were available for all to see. Charcot classified these symptoms into two broad categories of permanent physical defects like loss of sensation, impaired vision, or paralysis, and periodic fits, or 'convulsions', that arose spontaneously or when a patient was somehow distressed. He also identified clear stages to these fits, attempting to make sense of the disease in lieu of the biological evidence he anticipated.

Charcot documented his patients, employing the latest cutting-edge scientific equipment available to him – the camera – to photograph and categorise the postures the women took into patterns. The female body fainting listlessly backwards and the *arc-en-cercle* in which the hysterical patient sharply arches her back, leaving only the head and feet resting on the floor or bed, are two of the most famous postures defined by Charcot and his colleagues.[3] This technology elevated their findings, pandered to the new empiricism of the time that prized observable, objective evidence above all other forms of knowledge. The camera recorded what was there, and so provided 'objective' evidence for Charcot's patterns, reflecting a brain disease that would, he was certain, soon be discovered.

The Salpêtrière where Charcot worked wasn't just a living museum of pathology either, it was a theatre too.[4]

And Charcot had other tools in his scientific toolkit – like hypnosis, which he used to elicit the hysterical symptoms he wanted to categorise. Researchers reassured themselves that they weren't *evoking* performed behaviours from vulnerable patients, they were simply drawing out hysterical symptoms for long enough to allow for proper observation.

Charcot had many research subjects, some better known than others, and mainly women, and as he studied them, he began to see patterns in their postures and categorised them into types.

There was, however, something else his patients, and the many 'hysterics' to come, had in common, something that went overlooked by Charcot: a history of sexual abuse. It seems incredible now that a scientist – a neurologist, no less – would place such a premium on the shared symptoms displayed by his patients, but not the shared history. Then again, even today, trauma is frequently overlooked as a root of disorders. Even today, many psychiatrists still vastly prefer a biological, rather than experiential, explanation.

Louise Augustine Gleizes is the patient who skyrocketed Charcot to fame. What we know about Augustine was recorded by the doctor D.M. Bourneville who, alongside Charcot's photographer P. Regnard, recorded anything deemed 'noteworthy' about her case. She was fourteen when she first started seeing Charcot, and hadn't started her period yet, defying the belief at the time that hysteria could only come after menstruation.[5] Bourneville's notes describe Augustine as 'active, intelligent, affectionate, impressionable, temperamental', adding that she 'likes drawing attention to herself.'[6]

Augustine was tested with all the existing indicators of neurological conditions to see the difference in movement between the right and left side of her body. Charcot's methods included poking, prodding and administering drugs[7] – he was, after all, a neurologist, and every patient was simultaneously an experimental subject.[8] Traditional indicators were meticulously described, including temperature of various body parts, patterns of excretion, and of course, the ever-important marker of femininity, menstruation, once it started.[9]

A lack of mobility and sensation with no easily apparent underlying cause was one of the determining features for a diagnosis of hysteria. For Augustine, it was her right-hand side that was affected. She was numb in some parts and hypersensitive in others. She had also lost thought, vision and sense of colour[10] – all marks of hysteria. She also displayed the characteristic fainting fits common to so many of his patients, and so Charcot arrived at a diagnosis.

This is all documented in the official narrative. But if we scratch beneath the surface of this scientific case report, we get a different story. It is difficult to discern which details of Augustine's story were omitted, given that doctors were well convinced of the hysteric's tendencies to exaggerate and lie. From the notes, however, one salient theme is not difficult to believe: sexual harassment and assault.

Augustine grew up for the most part in a convent. While there, Augustine occasionally visited the wife of a decorator. The decorator was violent and on one occasion he hit his wife, tied her up by her hair, and then tried to rape Augustine.[11]

That summer, Augustine's mother took her to the house where she and her husband worked as servants. Augustine was told to call the man of the house 'Daddy' and to kiss him. At thirteen, she was removed from the convent and brought back to live with them. While there, 'Daddy' tried to have sex with her. She resisted and he failed the first few times. The third time he tried to seduce her, promised her gifts, then threatened her with a razor, forced her to drink alcohol, threw her on the bed and raped her. She bumped into 'Daddy' on the street sometime later and he grabbed her by the hair. She had a 'fit' after that.[12]

Shortly before her arrival at the hospital, Augustine was arguing a lot with her parents, who would scold her for her 'unladylike' behaviour. In one of these fights, she learned that her mother had been sleeping with her assaulter. She learned that her brother may even be his, and not her father's son. She realised that her mother may have brought her to the house as a proxy, or a gift.[13] She had discovered that she had been subjected to sexual assault and coercion as a pawn in adults' games.

These snippets give a sense of the texture of Augustine's life. The horrifying scenes of her rape would revisit her during hypnosis at the Salpêtrière – that's what made her such an 'alluring' star patient. And yet, as she rose to fame, with whole audiences gawking at her, no one thought to ask what the woman or girl with the body was trying to say.

Charcot and his followers built the basis for the science of hysteria by making a show of their patients. Charcot's lecture theatres became stages for performances beheld by students as well as an increasingly influential and international audience. Stage-lighting, iconographic art, enlarged photographs and costumes elevated the drama of his demonstrations. Women like Augustine who had been exposed to sexual assault were paraded around as part of an evasive taxonomy, bodies distilled into silent 'evidence' before trainee doctors or a public audience. Photographs were taken and displayed to taunt the public imagination with the threat of feral femininity. In Charcot's public lectures, hypnosis was often induced by ringing large gongs or tuning forks, or by applying electrical shock and pressure to 'hysterogenic' points on the body (typically the ovaries).[14] Augustine's memories and those of the numerous patients before and after her, became the evidence Charcot used to deduce his symptomology for a theory of a biological disease.

But when we take stock of Augustine's biography riddled with sexual threat and assault, the hysteric fits and visions start to seem less like symptoms of a problem situated within her, than an entirely proportionate response to physical and emotional violation. They seem more like embodied responses to traumatic events. And yet, Augustine's real experiences became irrelevant, were entirely erased, in the process of turning her body into evidence for the dysfunction of her mind.

The hysterical women did not just testify to the power of a new science. They also mirrored very particular gender roles. For Charcot, hysteria wasn't exclusive to women, but his patients were mainly women, and he made his name through his work with some legendary female patients. These women, their bodies and their postures, provided fertile ground for policing the bounds of what a woman should be. Female hysterics embodied many of the traits that had been conventionally associated with femininity – lability, fragility, susceptibility. At the same time, they enacted scenes of an often-sexual nature; unladylike behaviour that served as testament to their illness. Hysterical performances exemplified the fragility of women in general, while also pathologising these women in particular by drawing light to their gender transgressions. Audiences could gawk from a safe distance at the freakshow of feral femininity.

As well as being something of a spectator sport, hysterics in the nineteenth century proved useful models for oppression. During a time of social upheaval in France, against the backdrop of a fierce struggle between monarchy and secular republicans, the feminist movement was on the rise, sparking conservative anxieties about consolidating gender roles in a rapidly industrialising, strange, new, modern world. It is no coincidence that many of the traits Charcot used to describe hysterics, mirrored the language used to describe the feminists of the time, drawing a parallel that would serve to frame feminists as hysterics too. The feminist, like the hysteric, was either hyper-feminine – vain, malleable, suggestible, seductive – or not feminine enough – troublemaking, assertive, aggressive.

The science of hysteria presented the aims of women to leave the home and abandon their roles as babymakers, as unnatural and pathological, serving as 'a dramatic medical metaphor for everything that men found mysterious or unmanageable' in women, in the words of the medical historian Mark S. Micale.[15]

Charcot did not go unchallenged and was met with some criticism at the time, not least by feminists, for his condescension towards women; how he turned them into experimental subjects under the pretext of studying a disease for which he knew neither the cause nor the treatment,[16] guided only by the belief that the root cause had to be in their brains. Some scientists, too, questioned whether he was more of a showman than a scientist. The supposedly objective evidence Charcot was gathering by means of hypnosis, some claimed, was highly contrived, and did not represent discoveries but tricks. He had created the symptoms he purported to discover, they argued.

Eventually, Charcot's performance lost its audience.

The neurological evidence that was needed to support his supposedly scientific classifications, and to justify his method, did not come. Researchers were beginning to doubt whether hysteria had anything to do with the brain and nervous system at all.[17] And, slowly, a new interpretation of 'hysterical' behaviour emerged through the work of a neurologist from Vienna who had spent a few months studying at the hospital to learn from Charcot: Sigmund Freud.

Touching trauma

Freud's theory of hysteria came tantalisingly close to acknowledging the role that sexual violence continued to play in causing women's mental suffering – indeed, for a while it did – only in the end to fall short. Freud had been initially impressed by Charcot's approach, but he was also intrigued by the criticisms that suggested that Charcot had brought on the symptoms he purported to discover, and that there may be some other, non-biological basis to the disease to explore. In his early studies on the topic, he diverged from Charcot's neurological approach to make his mark on the debate and propose a different explanation.

In one study published in 1893, Freud showed hysterical symptoms, such as the 'paralysis' displayed by hysterical patients, to be entirely different to 'organic', physical paralysis caused by stroke or injury. Hysterical patients, he observed, did not move their paralysed limbs in ways that made anatomical sense[18]: a hysterical patient would drag her leg behind her, while someone organically paralysed would make a circumduction with the hip. Moreover, paralysis resulting from brain damage usually spared the hip area. Patients, he noted, seemed to move in a way that reflected a popular understanding of anatomy, rather than a medical one. These findings eventually led Charcot himself to abandon the physiological approach for one based on emotional trauma.[19] Charcot's findings suggested that there was more than simply something neurological going on, and Freud's observations raised the radical possibility that women were not suffering from neurological deficiencies, nor responding to the suggestions of their physicians, but perhaps had some other reason to behave this way.

One common thread that Freud noticed was that many hysterical women had experienced sexual trauma. Perhaps this was key to the cause of the disease.

But Freud soon hit the limits of his capacity to confront the violence of rape. The social implications were simply too great, and Freud became increasingly troubled by the prevalence of sexual assault among his female patients. Hysteria was so common among women that if his patients' stories were true, and if his theory was correct, he would be forced to conclude that 'perverted acts against children' were endemic, both among the proletariat in Paris, where he had first studied hysteria, and among the respectable bourgeois families of Vienna, where he had established his practice.[20] This was more than Freud's professional credibility could withstand, leaving only one solution – to stop listening to his female patients.[21] And so, Freud's theory, based on sexual trauma, gave way to another pathological version of femininity: that of sexual repression.

By 1987, Freud had fully replaced sexual exploitation with sexual repression as the 'locus' of hysteria.[22] He no longer believed that women's reports of sexual coercion and violence were memories of real events. They were, he asserted, actually remembered *fantasies* of sexual encounters from childhood. Memories of forbidden erotic feelings that we all shared, but that for some reason resurfaced in hysterical patients. Whatever had or hadn't happened to women was, to Freud, almost irrelevant, as the unconscious mind couldn't distinguish between fantasy and reality. The real problem, in any case, wasn't any sexual encounter, but femininity itself. Hysteria, he argued, was 'characteristically feminine',[23] the result of woman's inevitable lack.

'In a whole series of cases', he wrote in 1909, 'the hysterical neurosis is nothing but an excessive overaccentuation of the typical wave of repression through which the masculine type of sexuality is removed and the woman emerges.'[24] Freud now saw hysteria in relation to his all-important Oedipal theory. He posited that when young women find they lack a penis, they believe themselves to be castrated, leading to an inferiority complex, a form of internalised resentment towards other women, displayed as exaggerated emotional response. The concept of a 'castrated female' and their associated anxieties were what caused the nervous disposition of women, behaviour that enacts a lack, a void.[25] Women were always already physically scarred by the recognition of their own 'castration'[26] – in other words, by simply being women. For Freud, the scar that caused hysteria was still physical, but in a different sense to the belief that motivated Charcot. For Freud, hysteria was rooted in the lack of male genitalia, and *all* women suffered from this same lack.

Hysterical men

Between 1914 and 1915, as Freud was shoring up his theory of psychoanalysis that placed the roots of hysteria in sexual fantasies, the psychiatrist Charles Samuel Myers met three patients at the Duchess of Westminster's War Hospital in Le Touquet, France.[27] A war had broken out in Europe, sending thousands of young men into trenches, where they lived in appalling conditions, experienced prolonged bombardment, witnessed unprecedented scales of death, and lived with the constant threat of their own demise for months on end. [28] Some of these men were being sent from the battlefield with some peculiar symptoms. Myers had noticed some clear similarities between them.[29] The first of his patients was a twenty-year-old private, who had experienced shells bursting around him while he had been hooked by barbed wire (an eyewitness in the hospital reported that his escape was a 'sheer miracle'). This man had experienced some memory loss, but also impaired vision, smell and taste. The second patient, a corporal, aged twenty-five, reported he had been buried for eighteen hours due to a shell bursting and trapping him in the trench where he lay. He reports remembering nothing until he found himself in a dressing station at a barn lying on straw. He, too, had lost his vision, smell and taste. The third, a private aged twenty-three, was blown off a heap of bricks 15 feet high owing to a shell bursting close to him. He reasoned that he must have fallen into a pool of water, because he next remembered finding himself later that day in a cellar near a church with his clothes drenched. He didn't know how he left the cellar or who was there with him, but he remembered someone talking to him on a train and reminding him of being in the cellar. He lost his vision, smell and taste.[30] There were other symptoms, too, like shaking uncontrollably, dizziness, or sweating profusely. In short, these were very similar to the symptoms of hysteria.

There was nothing particularly unusual about these men, their temperaments, or their lives. But they shared a very clear, distinct experience of warfare. The symptoms were clearly not a response to sexual repression. They were uniquely diagnosed in men who had been at war, even if not all of them had experienced any obvious physical injury. Though the symptoms resembled hysteria, Myers reasoned that this had to be a distinct condition.

Myers coined a new term, *shell shock*, to describe the phenomenon he had observed in the soldiers,[31] and initially he believed it to have a biological cause: cerebral concussions and the rupture of small blood vessels resulting from proximity to the exploding shells, which the soldiers in his first case studies had in common. But it soon became clear that the same symptoms arose in soldiers not directly engaged in battle. This led Myers to distinguish 'shell concussion' (a neurological condition) from shell shock. Shell shock, slowly but surely, came to be understood as a psychological response to the extreme, traumatising conditions of war, as well as distinct from 'those whose disorder has a purely mental origin'. [32]

This would have come as a relief to the men who often faced hostility and ridicule on being sent from the front; public opinion, and the opinion of many psychiatrists, was that the symptoms of shell shock were simply tactics to exempt them from service, nothing more than shameful cowardice.

But research progressed to prove that shell shock was not a personal failing, but a response to traumatic experience. Abram Kardiner, an American psychiatrist who had studied under Freud, drew on psychoanalytic theory to coin the new condition of *war neurosis*. Kardiner saw how soldiers suffering from war neuroses often forgot the traumatic event itself, while at the same time behaving as if they were still in the midst of it. He viewed this combination of amnesia and physiological arousal as a mechanism to protect the ego integrity. Although he recognised that the similarities between war neuroses and hysteria – and indeed, most recognised that this was nothing more than a 'male hysteria'[33] – he was determined to make a distinction:

> When the word 'hysterical' ... is used, its social meaning is that the subject is a predatory individual, trying to get something for nothing. The victim of such neurosis is, therefore, without sympathy in court, and ... without sympathy from his physicians, who often take ... 'hysterical' to mean the individual is suffering from some persistent form of wickedness, perversity, or weakness of will.[34]

Male hysteria would not be associated with women or weakness, and instead would be a form of neuroses borne of difficult experience, rather than inherent inferiority.

The effort to protect the integrity of soldiers drew on a lineage of nineteenth-century efforts to understand men's physiological responses to war. The work of army surgeons had established that soldiers' distress was expressed through changes in the cardiovascular system. Arthur Myers coined the term *soldiers' heart* in 1870 to describe a disorder that included extreme fatigue, dyspnoea, palpitations, sweating, tremors, and occasionally complete syncope (fainting) often seen among soldiers involved in combat. In the next year, Jacob Mendez Da Costa, an army surgeon in the American Civil War, elaborated on Myers' work to define a condition variously called *irritable heart*, *effort syndrome*, and *Da Costa's syndrome*. In all cases, the symptoms these soldiers experienced were proposed to be a strictly biological response to the stress of battle.[35]

The movement this research reflected, in effect, was opposite to the one witnessed in the psychiatric response to hysteria. While hysteria was defined in the context of sexualised violence that many of these women had experienced, it soon evolved into a disorder that marked a deficiency in the women themselves; the sexual experiences came to be framed as by-the-by, possible figments of a defunctive woman's imagination. Soldiers' heart, on the other hand, functioned to protect a sense of male integrity by placing the cause of their biological experience with the conditions of war: the veritable opposite to 'it's all in your head'. As the psychiatrist Bessel van der Kolk put it, the explanation provided an 'honourable solution for all parties who might be compromised by people breaking down under stress: the soldier preserved his self-respect, the doctor did not have to diagnose personal failure or desertion, and military authorities did not have to explain psychological breakdowns in previously brave soldiers, or bother with troublesome issues such as cowardice, low unit morale, poor leadership, or the meaning of the war effort itself.'[36]

This explanation suited those in charge; and so, men at war preserved their dignity. Although with shell shock, like hysteria, it became established that there was a psychological component to the physiological responses of soldiers, soldiers' *experiences*, rather than their inherent failing, were still recognised as the cause. This is how the word 'trauma', previously exclusive to the field of surgery (trauma was first a medical term, used only to describe impact to the body),[37] came to be applied to the mind. Just as a bomb could sever your limbs, it could also rupture your mind.

Women's experience of war never got the same consideration. As men received a diagnosis to mark their experience of war appropriately as traumatic, there was a silence around the impact of the war on military nurses, many of whom were exposed to the same loss of autonomy, exhausting work in cramped conditions, constant bombardment and exposure to death and mutilation that soldiers were. As mothers, wives, widows or workers themselves, they experienced the effects of invasion, exodus, air raids or bereavement 'at home'. In addition, women experienced the trauma of their traumatised husbands returning home, and the domestic violence, directed at them, that this often precipitated. Yet the pain of women was not granted the legitimacy of shell shock. Female war 'neurosis' was only ever recognised outside official military discourse and medical forums. When it was acknowledged, this trauma was regarded as different in nature, with women being depicted as passive vessels of emotion awaiting news from the battlefield, and was never related to women's war service at home or abroad. Women themselves did not claim shell shock, either, even in the most harrowing descriptions of their experiences during the war and in its aftermath. It is probable that they did not see their own suffering as deserving of support, given the total lack of a publicly sanctioned language for their experience.[38] Long called hysterical, women had apparently internalised the view that their suffering reflected their deficiencies.

Doctors went to great pains to distinguish shell shock from hysteria. In doing so, they went some way in protecting men from the most damning judgements and repercussions thrown at them. While hysteria lives on in its various guises today, often diminishing the role of real events that precipitate mental distress for women, shell shock formed the foundations for a framework of understanding mental distress in the context of impactful events. That view was carried forward in the context of the other wars that followed. Concerned by the economic costs of psychiatric casualties during the First World War, the US military attempted to develop psychiatric screening methods to identify those who were psychologically unfit to withstand the demands of combat.[39] It soon became clear, though, that while some men might be more likely than others to develop psychological symptoms in the face of battle, no one was exempt from the impact of violence. These insights further spurred on a paradigm shift in psychiatry, towards recognising the role of the environment, rather than individual deficiency, in causing mental and physiological symptoms. These insights, along with new research into the protective effects of the relationships among soldiers against the impact of war, drove a decisive shift away from psychoanalytic theories about the inner causes of mental deviation, and towards the interactions between individuals and their environments.

By the 1960s, new ideas from the social and behavioural sciences were being integrated into medicine, leading to new concepts, like stress, that recognised the impact that experiences have on minds. Clinicians and researchers studying and caring for a range of groups, from Holocaust survivors to rape victims, battered children to Vietnam veterans, developed discrete pockets of knowledge about the effects of particular forms of psychological trauma,[40] and in the 1970s, researchers started to integrate this knowledge. These changes were spurred along by the lobbying of Vietnam War veterans who had returned from war to an underequipped Veterans Administration (V. A.). Veterans, their families, and a new wave of interest among mental health professionals in trauma, all campaigned for a new diagnosis that grouped together 'civilian' and 'military' trauma response syndromes under the label of PTSD. In 1980, PTSD was introduced into the DSM-III – the third edition of psychiatry's manual of disorders.[41]

The introduction of PTSD was a landmark in psychiatry,[42] demarcating a space in which mental distress could be discussed, even within the medical parameters of the DSM, as something that happened *to you*, and not as some form of dysfunction *in you*. And, while the traumatic experiences more common to women than men were included in this category, the understanding of the symptoms of PTSD and appropriate treatment were developed largely in the context of war, predominantly among soldiers, who were mainly men. To this day, it is taking a long time for the psychiatric institution, and culture at large, to give the same credence to the experiences that disproportionately traumatise women, as war has done men.

Interpersonal violence

As we have explored, there are various forms of trauma not experienced in combat. Freud and Charcot's patients had experienced violence of a different nature to the soldiers Myer and Kardiner observed. Women then, and now, are less likely to meet the violence on the public stage of the battlefield, as they are the violence that happens in the privacy of the home. The patterns of gendered violence are by now familiar to researchers, and population studies have repeatedly confirmed the same findings. Consistently, men more often report physical attacks, combat experience, and being threatened with a weapon, held captive, or kidnapped as the cause of trauma, while women report predominantly interpersonal violence: rape, sexual molestation, childhood parental neglect, and childhood physical abuse.[43] Global estimates by the World Health Organisation suggest 1 in 3 women will experience physical or sexual violence in her lifetime, most often by an intimate partner.[44] Women are also more likely than men to be survivors of child sexual abuse; in the UK, an astonishing 25 per cent of girls, compared to 18 per cent of boys aged 13 to 17 have reported having experienced some form of physical violence in an intimate relationship.[45] There is also a larger sex difference for severe and repeated abuse – in 75 per cent of domestic violence and abuse-related crimes the victim is female, and the disparity is the same for victims of domestic homicide.[46] Globally, sexual abuse is the most common form of trauma for women, eclipsing the effects of other forms of physical abuse or neglect, war, terrorism, community violence, or accidents.[47]

The effects of exposure to traumatic events also differs between genders; understandable, of course, considering the very different nature of the experiences involved. Women are twice as likely as men to develop PTSD following exposure to interpersonal violence, compared to the forms of violence men more commonly experience.[48] This makes sense, considering that the interpersonal violence women experience is distressing and destabilising in multiple and complex ways. This kind of trauma is shrouded in secrecy and shame from the onset. Given that attacks often happen in the context of close relationships, victims and survivors have to deal with a sense of betrayal, a disruption of their basic trust in people, and of who they thought they were in relation to those people. It is uniquely destabilising as it undercuts the structures that are supposed to provide safety, belonging, and identity. Unlike the event of war, that undeniably exposes people to unfathomable distress, soldiers can return home, can maintain a safe distance from the events that traumatised them, and are more likely to find a safe context in which to recover their sense of self. The enemy, in war, is out there; the victims and survivors of interpersonal violence find themselves often having to recover in the same context as that in which they faced the traumatising violence, while also no longer able to make sense of the notion of a home when all sense of safety and predictability has been pulled from under their feet. Fearing that speaking out will expose them to further danger, they are met by a culture that easily dismisses rape allegations and protects perpetrators. In the wake of violence, while still facing the ongoing threat, the victims and survivors of interpersonal violence are likely to have their distrust in others reinforced in a world that doesn't support them. The terror of this kind of isolation, the chronic and ongoing insecurity experienced in the persistence of this kind of threat, is unique to the interpersonal violence predominantly experienced by women. And so, rape is associated with the highest conditional probability of developing PTSD for both men and women.[49] Women develop PTSD twice as often as men do because they are more frequently exposed to interpersonal trauma. Only prisoner-of-war experiences carry a similar risk of PTSD.[50] And it makes sense that interpersonal trauma shakes people to the core precisely because it doesn't happen on the frontline.

Trauma is a term that is often thrown about quite loosely, but what does it actually mean here; what are the actual impacts on people's lives? In the language of psychiatry, we know that intimate partner violence is associated with a threefold increase of a psychiatric diagnosis.[51] Women who have been abused by a partner are more likely to have a diagnosis of depression, anxiety, schizophrenia or bipolar disorder than other women.[52] All these psychological problems are entwined with, reinforce, and are reinforced by, physical problems. Victims of abuse, whether sexual in nature or not, suffer increased levels of chronic headaches, gastrointestinal disorders, heart problems, gynaecological problems, abdominal pain, as well as chronic stress-related central nervous system and immune system dysfunction, leading to elevated risk of everything from HIV to asthma.[53] Let alone their greatly elevated risk of suicide.[54]

These correlations give a crude idea of the impact of this particular kind of violence on an individual life. They lead to different questions about the experience of women formerly diagnosed with hysteria; questions about what happened to them, how they learned to cope, and how they can begin to feel safe enough to change their coping mechanisms. They do not lead to questions about biological brokenness. When we begin to validate and give serious attention to the trauma women disproportionately face, we begin to find explanations that come closer to those we have historically given to men.

Complex trauma

PTSD should have been an opportunity to revise our understanding of psychological suffering, not just for men, but for people in general. Had psychiatrists turned their attention to the particular experiences shared by women, as well as men, they may have developed a more comprehensive and relevant understanding of the impact of trauma on women much earlier on. But women were excluded from these explanations. And so, survivors of sexual abuse, activists, and psychiatrists too, have had to push for a more complete theory of trauma, to include the impact of the violence on women.

Given the particular difficulties people who experience interpersonal violence face, many mental health professionals have argued that the framework of PTSD, originally and predominantly developed to describe the experience of men at war, does not adequately describe or address the trauma of interpersonal violence predominantly experienced by women in the home.

The American psychiatrist Judith Herman was one of the first to ask whether PTSD captured the experience of traumatised women. In her seminal 1992 book *Trauma and Recovery*, she drew on her extensive clinical work with incest survivors and on the role of childhood trauma in borderline personality disorder,[55] to make what should really have been an obvious point: that responses to trauma will differ according to the nature, severity, and timescale of traumatic events. Herman argued that human trauma response should be understood as a spectrum.[56] At one end is the kind of acute stress reaction that resolves on its own without treatment, and on the other end, a form of what she called, 'complex post-traumatic stress disorder' that results from the kind of trauma of prolonged or repeated abuse. Classic PTSD would exist somewhere between these two. Herman worked alongside other psychiatrists, including Bessel van der Kolk, to have complex PTSD included in the DSM. Initially, in 1993, the American Psychiatric Association's PTSD committee agreed, and voted to add complex PTSD to the next version of the DSM. Yet it did not appear in the 1994 edition, the DSM-IV, and it hasn't been included since.

Initially, the committee considered including complex PTSD under the category of 'disorders of extreme stress not otherwise specified (DESNOS)' but eventually rejected the idea. DESNOS encompassed some important criteria that capture the specificity of the trauma resulting from interpersonal violence. It included, for example, the criteria of 'alterations in relationships to others, such as not being able to trust, not being able to feel intimate with people'. This is different from some of the superficially similar criteria used to describe the impact of trauma on relationships under PTSD in the current DSM. These criteria include 'Feelings of detachment or estrangement from others', or 'Persistent, disordered cognitions about the cause or consequences of traumatic event(s) that lead the individual to blame himself/herself or others', or 'Persistent and exaggerated negative beliefs or expectations about oneself, others, or the world (e.g. 'I am bad', 'No one can be trusted', 'The world is completely dangerous', 'My whole nervous system is permanently ruined'). These do not adequately capture how interpersonal violence disrupts someone's sense of safety and security in their relationships and home. The last criteria, in particular, could even be misconstrued if applied to someone currently experiencing interpersonal trauma, as the threat of repeated violence could very well be real. A person with complex PTSD could still be experiencing abuse at home and may not feel ready or safe enough to discuss it; there is nothing exaggerated about this view. When the nature of interpersonal violence is not understood, survival strategies can be pathologised as symptoms of a disorder, as they were for Charcot's hysterics.

All this would have come to light much sooner, if psychiatry had embraced PTSD as an important revision to its theories of hysteria that, at various moments in time, had rooted mental distress either in the body, or the personality.

But the resistance we saw in Freud's time to recognising women's trauma persists. It wasn't until 2018 that the World Health Organisation finally included complex PTSD in the 11th revision of its International Classification of Diseases (ICD-11), a psychiatric manual like the DSM that is used most commonly outside of the US. This edition was published in line with a new public health perspective that emphasises what is clinically useful to patients,[57] and has directed research into treatment that is appropriate for this specific form of trauma. Accordingly, the most relevant research in the area has come from the UK and Germany, rather than the US, which continues to cling to old definitions.

I had the privilege of speaking with Herman, who detailed to me the nature of the resistance she faced from the DSM committee in her early work in getting complex PTSD recognised:

> The argument was interesting. They said it overlapped with too many other disorders: affective disorders, personality disorders, dissociative disorders, somatisation disorders, and addictions. And I just thought, *Yeah, that's the point*. [laughs] You don't want people making one or other of those diagnoses and missing the central issue. That's how you end up with polypharmacy or inadequate treatment because you're only treating the depression or the addiction, or you've diagnosed someone with borderline personality disorder but you

haven't asked about trauma. But I think it impinged on too many people's turf.

The overlap noted by the members of the DSM committee, between complex PTSD and so many other diagnoses, should have indicated the centrality of trauma to so many of the mental experiences currently treated as psychiatric disorders. But, as ever, the profession's legitimacy was at stake. Complex PTSD challenged the carefully guarded expertise of a profession, alongside the types of explanations that place the origins of women's distress in the brain or personality. In fact, PTSD itself had already challenged this dominant view, by positing experience, rather than biology, as the cause of distress in men. But complex PTSD goes even further, in describing the specific texture of that impact in the context of a certain type of experience. In short, it is speaking a different language; one based on outside factors, rather than the classification of biological disease that has been so essential to the particular form of medical legitimacy psychiatrists have sought since the age of Enlightenment science. Complex PTSD raises the spectre of the question that psychiatrists have long ignored, about how psychiatry factors trauma into its explanations for psychiatric disease, when it has built itself as a science akin to medicine that looks for explanations in brains, rather than the experiences people endure.

Given the shame and fear that prevents many from reporting interpersonal violence, it is essential that they are equipped with the appropriate tools to protect themselves and then heal from these experiences. These may not be medical at all. The criteria for PTSD in the DSM stipulate that symptoms must occur after the 'traumatic event'. But interpersonal violence, such as abuse and manipulation, is not an 'event', but an ongoing barrage; much like the ongoing attacks soldiers in the trenches faced, but with none of the public recognition or protection, nor the possibility of distance from the ongoing threat. Real threats require social support and real protection. People facing real threats require safety before therapy. Then, they require ongoing mental health support to make sense of their experiences, and to *feel* safe again. A diagnosis can help individuals and others recognise the severity of the impact of these forms of structural violence, but it is not in itself a solution.

The debates about the severity and nature of the trauma faced by the women who have suffered interpersonal violence is not just a debate for psychiatrists, but a debate about whose trauma we recognise as a society. Over a decade after the First World War supposedly awakened psychiatry to the impact of experiences on human minds, the particular threats women face in the world out there are still often framed as a psychiatric problem that exists in her. Today, hysteria continues to be diagnosed in women under a new guise, with 'Hysteria' disappearing unceremoniously from the DSM in 1980. But while the word had ceased, the concept hadn't. Women were no longer hysterical, but *histrionic*. Scratch beneath this modern gloss and you'd find the same old hysteria in its latest guise of histrionic personality disorder (or HPD). It wasn't the end of hysteria; it was simply a new word for it.

According to the DSM today, this disorder might present in a variety of ways. An individual with HPD might be uncomfortable when not the centre of attention, display inappropriate sexually seductive or provocative behaviour, express rapidly shifting and shallow emotions, use physical appearance to draw attention to themselves, speak in an excessively impressionistic way that is lacking in detail, behave dramatically, with exaggerated expression of emotion, be easily influenced by others or circumstances, and consider relationships to be more intimate than they actually are.[58]

This set of behaviours, of which a patient must display at least five to satisfy a diagnosis of HPD, is a familiar caricature. Describing behaviour that still has the taste of Charcot's patients' performativity, the histrionic is impressionable, labile, suggestible – too feminine – and at the same time egocentric and narcissistic – freakishly masculine. The prevalence of HPD in the population has remained fairly stable over time.[59] Women continue to be diagnosed with HPD about 4 times more frequently than men, and research has shown that psychiatrists are much more likely to apply the diagnosis to women because it evokes a feminine stereotype.[60] There is a marked lack of literature of HPD compared to other disorders included in the same category of personality disorders characterised by unpredictable and dramatic behaviour in the DSM, which also includes Anti-Social (ASPD), Borderline (BPD), and Narcissistic (NPD). As for so many conditions perceived to affect predominantly women, it seems to follow that HPD is less worthy of investment and serious attention. No wonder people diagnosed with HPD often suffer from depression and experience panic attacks.[61] This is a very normal response to having your real problems dismissed and reframed as a pathology.

That hysteria still exists as a disease in the DSM is problematic for those diagnosed with it (HPD is diagnosed in about 0.9 per cent of the general population globally). The label is problematic because it likely obscures the real nature of this group's distress. It is also problematic because, as we have seen, psychiatric diagnoses aren't just medical tools but are ideas that pervade culture. As long as we continue to sanction hysteria with the ever-authoritative language of science, we give legitimacy to people and institutions that leverage psychiatric diagnoses against women. We give legitimacy to courts that can use HPD to refute a woman's words in a rape trial, or to justify barring a woman's access to custody, parental rights and welfare. We legitimise the public figures who use misogyny to gain support, or anyone who dismisses a woman on the grounds of her being 'hysterical'. This scientific failing is also a cultural failing that reinforces the oppression of women in society at large.

Years of contestation have followed the various revisions to the DSM's classification.[62] The critiques centre around how unspecific the HPD profile is, which has always been the case with a diagnosis of hysteria. The critics of modern HPD argue how the same multiple and contradictory misogynistic binds perpetuate the same ideas about femininity that prevent women from being taken seriously everywhere. Despite its shaky empirical grounds, however, women continue to be diagnosed with and treated for the condition. While the first line of treatment is supposed to be psychotherapy, psychiatrists often turn to drugs; rather than pursuing real solutions, psychiatry chooses to subdue.

Women still lack a socially sanctioned or credible language, or support – granted to men – for the traumas they experience. We continue to live in a society and in communities that too willingly condone violence at varying levels of severity against women. When we decide, collectively, that interpersonal violence is real violence, when we give credence to the trauma experienced by women at home, we draw into public awareness the societal changes that are necessary for recovery. Addressing trauma, properly, is centrally about deconstructing the gendered binaries that stratify trauma and experience in the social world.

The issue of trauma shows us forcefully that social change is a prerequisite for mental recovery, because the divisions that delineate the public and the private also sever the sane from the insane, the credible from the uncredible, the heard from the silenced, the persons granted dignity and rights from those deemed subhuman, broken or criminal. There are no shortcuts, and while we need to do what we can to secure our individual survival in an imperfect society, real recovery will have to happen in the context of collective responsibility.

It is time for HPD to join hysteria in the annals of bygone diagnoses. We have to reach for alternatives that validate women's experiences, however imperfect these new tools might still be. We do, however, need to look to that archive to remind us of a history that still illuminates the sexist dismissals in culture and psychiatry today, to bring to light the subtler misogyny that characterises the use of many of the diagnoses we will discuss in this book. We will need the history to arm us with a vigilance to how hysteria appears in new guises to dismiss and discredit women today.

As long as we continue to leverage hysteria, the real problem remains unnamed; as long as we diagnose sexual repression rather than sexual abuse; as long as we diagnose femininity like a disease, instead of tackling the problems women face; as long as we cast reaction as overreaction, we are re-enacting this societal abuse. In all but name, the disease of hysteria persists, and despite its 'disappearance' from the DSM, hysteria remains untreated.

When we place hysteria in the context of the history of responses to trauma, we see the real problems it has obscured and erased from psychiatry. We also see, though, that a different interpretation, and a response that takes traumatic experiences seriously, is possible.

2

A Billion-Dollar Industry

As the history of hysteria and PTSD shows us, psychiatry, for a while at least, abandoned its biological roots. The official psychiatric explanations of mental distress that emerged through the early and mid-1900s were largely not based on the neurological explanations of mental suffering like Charcot's. Especially after the Second World War, psychoanalytic theories, like Freud's, emphasised how experiences shaped a person's inner world. These explanations had proven, through the war, to be more useful in understanding the symptoms of trauma, for one. They explained mental distress as an inner conflict, often connected to stunted childhood development. The target of therapies was a person's psyche, not their neurology.

The role of context, like violence and abuse, wasn't always included in this approach to mental distress, but a social understanding did grow around it. The years after the Second World War saw a real shift among leading American psychiatrists, whereby social problems were, perversely, pinned on the psychological problems of individuals. Psychiatry became central to tackling everything from the appeal of authoritarian governments to anti-Semitism, poverty and social deviance, crime, and social unrest.[1] New professions appeared, like social workers, who worked alongside psychiatrists, reflecting the link between social conditions and the state of people's minds. As dubious as it might be to think of social problems as the result of individual failings, drawing the link between people's mental wellbeing and the social world around them did lay the groundwork for a new approach to alleviating mental suffering that helped people with the real problems they faced. Many of these psychiatrists and mental health workers argued vehemently against the medical approaches to treating mental disease that targeted bodies and brains, like electrotherapy and surgeries. These could never be treatments in their own rights, and had to be administered alongside psychotherapy and psychosocial interventions.[2]

There was a similar envisioned use for the drugs, like the antidepressants, that appeared in the 1950s. These, some psychiatrists argued, could be used as tools to get people out of psychiatric hospitals, and into the community. They weren't cures, but aids that could sufficiently stabilise people to get them back to living. Their appearance became the justification for a programme that came to be known as 'deinstitutionalisation'. This programme, which was launched under the president John F. Kennedy in the US in the 1960s, failed dramatically. Drugs without the accompanying social support, couldn't deliver even on the limited aim to stabilise people. Without help, medicated patients struggled to reintegrate into society. Drugs turned out to have such significant side effects that many patients, once they were released from the hospital, decided to stop taking them. Many ex-hospital patients lived in substandard for-profit boarding houses with insufficient healthcare, on the streets, or in jails. Some lucky ones were forced to move in with their parents, who in turn felt unsupported by the state, and were becoming increasingly weary and angry.[3]

As the century progressed, critiques of psychiatry's early methods mounted. Various activist movements pointed to the power vested in psychiatry's definitions of insanity. Feminism, a growing movement, started to reveal the fabric of sexual abuse connecting many of the supposed complexes psychoanalysts identified in female patients. Gay people, too, launched a systematic critique, and protested against having their sexual and romantic preferences pathologised.[4] Other survivor groups, some part of a growing movement known as 'anti-psychiatry' argued against psychiatry's methods of punishment and control, claiming that many of these aimed to manage social deviance, more than they helped people.[5] Transcultural, or cultural, psychiatry also emerged in the 1950s, showing that our ideas of insanity are defined by a particular cultural context: for example, what might be considered a trance state and a visit from an ancestral spirit in some African and African-American cultures, might be interpreted as a symptom of psychosis according to the diagnostic schemes of western psychiatry. The critiques of psychiatry amassed. Even health insurance companies started to doubt psychiatrists' competence and, in the midst of a recession in mid-1970s America, questioned why they should reimburse clinicians who weren't even real doctors.[6]

By the 1980s, psychiatry was a profession in crisis. In the midst of the affront of criticisms, the voices of psychiatrists who favoured a biological approach, grew stronger. They argued that their late nineteenth-century predecessors had been on the right track, and that the hope for the profession, and so its patients, lay in biological, more properly scientific, rather than fluffy psychoanalytic, methods. This is how the profession decided it would redeem its legitimacy and also differentiate itself from the hordes of new mental health workers taking over the field of psychotherapy: clinical social workers, psychiatric nurses, counsellors and clinical psychologists. It was time for a paradigm shift.

The return to a biological approach was reflected in the discipline's diagnostic guide. In 1980, the American Psychiatric Association (APA) radically revised the third edition of the Diagnostic and Statistical Manual of Mental Disorders (DSM). The manual was supposed to offer a standardised guideline for diagnosing and treating mental conditions but, in practice, diagnostic decisions varied widely between practitioners. The diagnostic criteria were too vague. The APA decided to aim for a more robust system of classification. It would root its definitions and classifications firmly in biology, replacing the psychoanalytic with biological language and concepts, based on the latest research.[7]

These biological psychiatrists blamed psychoanalysis for their own field's waning influence. Back in the early 1900s, Freud and his followers had derailed what they saw as a perfectly credible neurological approach to understanding mental distress. The truth was, of course, that biological approaches had actually fallen short of helping people with experiences linked to trauma. The developments that did target bodies rather than a person's psyche, hadn't proven to be anywhere near to stand-alone solutions. Techniques like electrotherapy were considered increasingly controversial, and the psychotropic drugs that appeared from the 1950s onwards were considered aids mitigating symptoms, but not complete solutions to helping people get back on their feet, especially after the failed project of deinstitutionalisation.

Now, though, many psychiatrists claimed, new developments in neuroscience, genetics and drugs were the key; this time, they would prove that mental disorders were brain diseases. With it would come cures, not just aids to recovery. These claims weren't built on any real scientific advancement, but on a decision to establish psychiatry as a biological science. The evidence was still to come.

The decade of the brain

With the revision of the DSM, the 1980s saw a renewed interest in biological, and specifically neurological, research, returning to the hope of early psychiatrists like Charcot that neurology alone could explain mental suffering. But the idea that the mysteries of mental disorders can be resolved by a deeper understanding of the brain really took flight in the 1990s.[8] This interest was accompanied by the question of how a more direct study of the brain could illuminate psychological phenomena. The study of the brain and nervous system, now known as neuroscience, was increasingly discussed within and beyond biomedicine as representing an optimistic future of medical discovery, with then-US President George H. W. Bush signing a presidential declaration committing the 1990s to be the 'Decade of the Brain'.[9] The statement signalled the growth of neuroscience, as well as the future benefits to be gained from this cutting-edge field.[10] It also formed part of a larger effort involving the Library of Congress and the National Institute of Mental Health of the National Institutes of Health (NIH) 'to enhance public awareness of the benefits to be derived from brain research'.[11]

The announcement was followed by a sizeable increase in the visibility of neuroscience.[12] Brain research was more widely publicised in relation to the new government aims, but also through various national awareness-raising campaigns, the increased visibility of advocacy groups for individual diseases, and a massive media interest in breakthroughs in neuroscience.[13] Scientists flocked to the discipline,[14] many from molecular biology and computer science, introducing new cutting-edge techniques to the world of psychiatry, such as functional imaging and molecular genetics. A strong alliance developed between congressional leaders, the administration, representatives of disease advocacy groups, scientists themselves, and leaders at the NIH in promoting neuroscience.[15]

The decade of the brain continued into the new millennium. Brain science had yet to deliver on its potential to explain psychiatric disease, but the hope in its potential for human health remained strong. The NIH remained determined to stimulate innovation in this field.[16] In 2005, they decided to focus on fostering closer partnerships between universities and companies. This pipeline would ensure that neuroscientific research findings would make their way efficiently from the laboratory bench to the patient's bedside in the form of medical products, including diagnostics, medicines, and technologies. Elias Zerhouni, NIH director at the time, wrote that the model would lead to revolutionary transformations in human health:

> It is the responsibility of those of us involved in today's biomedical research enterprise to translate the remarkable scientific innovations we are witnessing into health gains for the nation. In order to address this imperative, we at the National Institutes of Health (NIH) asked ourselves: What novel approaches can be developed

that have the potential to be truly transforming for human health?[17]

Zerhouni paints the NIH as generous custodians, bestowing the gift of health on society through scientific innovation. 'Health' was becoming an ever-shinier word. In the biomedical era, the tools of medicine were increasingly discussed by policymakers as solutions to problems that in previous eras may have been regarded as the realm of social policy, like care provision or housing. Governments increasingly prioritised treating the poor health of people (often caused by societal neglect), rather than improving their living conditions. Today, we continue to place a lot of hope in medical solutions to improve our health. While we improve our lifestyles and buy the wellbeing products that might help us maximise our health as a matter of routine, there is always the hope that, for serious conditions, medicine will come to the rescue with a cure. Health is the glittering final frontier for the nation, and scientific innovation is framed as *the* path there. The potential gains are so great, it would be almost immoral not to pursue them.

While the translation pipeline was supposedly about human health, it also generated healthy profits. Starting in 2006, the NIH grew a nationwide network of academic, so-called clinical translational science centres focused on optimising research programmes and environments in order to push neuroscience research towards clinical applications.[18] This set-up was incredibly conducive to commercialisation. The new centres provided a pathway for investors, as well as pharmaceutical and biotechnology companies, to create partnerships with universities and university laboratories, enabling biopharmaceutical companies to outsource the riskiest parts of early-stage neuroscience innovation to non-profit universities. University research teams became small biotechnology start-ups and external industry partners became early-stage investment firms.[19] All this to ensure a steady flow of medical products from universities to companies, and a steady flow of new tools from companies to labs, to speed up this medical production line.

The NIH spent over $5 billion between 2005 and 2018 on grants through just its science award programme.[20] The proponents of translational research continued to justify this expenditure with the ever-imminent promise of optimised, widespread health. These words are hard to argue with. And usually, we don't. The promise of medical innovation has long been the hope on psychiatry's horizon. The promise of medical research has been a currency of our time, and, since the decade of the brain, most of that hope has been vested in the potential of brain research. And, of course, profit and wellbeing aren't necessarily mutually exclusive – financial flows are the animating engine of medical research. And yet, the language of health and hope is disingenuous when money and profit have become more than an enabler, and instead the driving force for research, regardless of the evidence.

Today, the translational pipeline determines what is 'good' science and what is not. If academic findings can be translated into marketable outcomes, like a new antidepressant, or diagnostic technology, they are deemed more important, considered a 'win' for human health, often even before they have been proven to be useful to patients, or scientifically rigorous. This system for creating wealth circumvents the very important question of the use these medical products hold for people themselves, in clinical practice, as well as the very fundamental question, never addressed in the rhetoric of brain science, of whether this is the most helpful form of innovation for societies at all.

Profit, in a profit-driven system, is often conflated with progress. When we look at the reality of the state of the field, the investments and industry partnerships that supposedly signalled hope for the future of the field, were actually a response to a dearth of useful studies. Profit tends to run away with itself, with little regard for the value lost in the pursuit of financial growth over human care.

The birth of big pharma

In 1997, the FDA weakened its regulations over direct-to-consumer marketing, and the brain-based theory of mental distress took on a new life of its own. If mental disorders existed in the brain as diseases, they would need medical solutions: antidepressants and anti-anxiety medication, all of which could be profited from. During the decade of the brain, clinicians and academic researchers became intimately involved in the marketing required to sustain a rapidly expanding market for biomedical cures to mental disease. The marketing strategies employed by companies in this set-up was both innovative and aggressive. Researchers were paid sizeable sums to perform studies and promote drugs to colleagues at conferences; when these experts did not secure the soaring prescriptions expected of them, their contracts were unceremoniously aborted.[21] Drug companies also formed alliances with family advocacy groups that supported the medical model of mental illness, because this was one of the most effective ways of winning over patients. When the FDA relaxed its regulations on advertising for prescription drugs, psychiatric drugs quickly became one of the most heavily advertised drugs, and continue to be so even today.[22]

Particularly in the US, companies took to advertising to educate people in the supposed biological facts of depression that only drugs could fix.[23] Amidst all this, Pfizer was the first to base a direct-to-consumer ad campaign specifically on the idea that depression was caused by a deficiency of certain biochemicals in the brain – a 'chemical imbalance'. Early print ads for Zoloft included a cartoon of neurons emitting neurotransmitters before and after treatment.[24]

There emerged a new paradigm for making sense of mental disorder, so common today we take it for granted: whatever experiences a person has that might cause them distress, these affect us via the brain, and therefore the most direct way to treat people with mental distress is by targeting the brain, via medication. This all sounds so intuitive now, because it has been the dominant narrative since the 1980s. But it is by no means a given that brain mechanisms cause mental distress. To talk of brains in relation to mental disorders might make sense; they are involved, of course, in psychosis or anxiety or depression, but this does not imply that they are the cause of mental experience. Brains mediate our experience of the world, and any mental experience arises through an interaction of a person, including their neural circuits, with their environment; but we cannot argue that experiences are simply projections of the neural circuits in our heads. This would be a reductive view that eviscerates and demotes the crucial role of the environment we are in. We are not brains in vats, after all.

Nonetheless, the new DSM corroborated this view of mental disorder. While the first and second editions of the

DSM had still drawn on quite old, psychoanalytic concepts of 'mental disorder' as a universal human capacity influenced by social factors like unconscious drives, early childhood experiences and family dynamics,[25] the new DSM defined mental diseases as heritable brain diseases: as discrete, molecular mechanisms that were distinct from normal, healthy brains. The implication was, again, that these were biological entities that could be identified and targeted with the right drugs.

The new explanations were useful, of course, to psychiatrists staking their claim to the territory of mental health by protecting their exclusive drug-prescribing rights. Only they, with their medical training, could responsibly prescribe in the best interest of patients, they argued.[26]

And yet, in a familiar refrain to the history of medicalised psychiatry, there was no evidence that companies were delivering on the hope they would bring to the lives of patients. The 1990s and early 2000s were, on the contrary, a 'barren time for the discovery of novel drugs for psychiatric disorders', in the words of one *Nature Review* article.[27] The best this period of innovation managed to deliver in terms of treatments was slight improvements to drugs that had already been in use since the 1950s, such as the new selective serotonin reuptake inhibitor antidepressants (SSRIs), and new antipsychotics like clozapine. In December 1987, the FDA approved the pharmaceutical company Eli Lilly's SSRI as an antidepressant. Its name would become emblematic of an era of unprecedented levels of medically sanctioned drug use: Prozac. SSRIs caused fewer of the short-term side effects but they did not work better than older drugs, and definitely not for everyone, and as time went on, their long-term, harmful health effects, including vomiting and loss of appetite, and even a higher risk of suicide, became searingly clear.[28] And yet psychiatric drug sales boomed.[29]

Drugs for diseases

Prozac, like SSRIs, is today almost synonymous with the term 'antidepressant'. It is one of the most widely used drugs of its kind, although it is not just prescribed for depression, but also for a range of other disorders including OCD, anxiety, bulimia, panic disorder, and PMDD. In 2021, it was the 25th most commonly prescribed drug in the United States, with around 23 million prescriptions, only preceded by medications largely targeting physiological conditions like high blood pressure, diabetes, digestive and respiratory issues, along with a few other antidepressants.[30]

Prozac was, and continues to be, marketed as a drug to target a chemical imbalance of serotonin in the brain. Serotonin had begun to be investigated by various international teams in the hope of developing an antidepressant that would avoid the cardiovascular side effects that had been associated with other antidepressants thus far, notably benzodiazepines, that worked less selectively.[31] Researchers had noted that the chemicals that were effective in lifting moods also seemed to block the brain's serotonin reuptake mechanisms.[32] And so came the earliest attempts at manufacturing what today are known as selective serotonin reuptake inhibitors (SSRIs).

Prozac sales boomed. Clinicians preferred prescribing Prozac to other drugs on the market, because it was considered a safer, 'clean' drug, and for that same reason, they were liberal with their prescriptions: they prescribed it even for patients with milder symptoms of depression, or, given one of the drug's welcome side effects, for weight loss.[33] Enthusiasm for Prozac continued to grow as its applications continued to bleed over the margins of its intended function as an antidepressant. In 1993, the psychiatrist Peter Kramer published a book called *Listening to Prozac*, in which he drew on his patients' stories to suggest that Prozac didn't just correct but also enhanced people's personalities. More than lifting depression, he described how people became 'improved': clearheaded, confident, relaxed; how they felt more attractive, advanced their careers, made more friends. One example of a woman who used the drug to advance her career, made Kramer so bold as to claim that Prozac was a 'feminist' drug.[34] Prozac held the potential not just for radical personal transformation, it seemed, but for societal transformation (all, conveniently, while doing nothing to change social structures at all). Kramer predicted a future of 'cosmetic psychopharmacology', in which antidepressants were prescribed to give social confidence to the shy, to brighten dull personalities, to give employees the confidence they needed to climb the corporate ladder.[35] His words turned out to be prophetic; but what he missed were the harmful implications of this vision of pharmaceutically fuelled self-improvement.

The consequence of the view reflected in Kramer's gradually realised vision, is that the division between truly pathological and economically sub-optimal became increasingly blurred. Prozac is prescribed for a personality boost, and shyness is suddenly a phobia. Pathology is economically defined. Mental distress – just like economic advancement in today's climate – is framed as an individual responsibility rather than a societal one, and biological psychiatry continues to push this narrative by locating problems in brains rather than social systems.[36]

The personality-enhancing function of Prozac was able to coexist with the idea that this was a medication specifically designed to target a medical condition known as depression. And this was possible due to an unwavering belief in the biological narrative that could flexibly stand in for multiple stories, about the origins of madness in the brain, or as a deviation from productivity. And while some critics drew attention to the fictions that connected the aim to 'fix' people and the claims to be able to fix all their problems with a simple pill, in the year of Kramer's book's publication, Prozac sales increased by 15 per cent.[37]

Diseases for drugs

During the first half of the 1990s, Prozac took the western world by storm. Marketing efforts had turned the pill into the perfect emblem of productivity, optimising and enhancing modern-day workers. Marketing innovation for these blockbuster antidepressants, which were followed by other similarly flashy medications, repeatedly outstripped scientific progress, fuelling a steadily growing market. In the second half of the decade, however, patents started to expire. And so, drug companies turned to a new market-expanding strategy: new markets would emerge with new diseases, so why not invent a few? This was where the true innovation happened, as SSRI-producing companies began the hunt for an array of culturally resonant diagnoses to market their drugs for, in a process the psychiatrist Donald Klein has referred to as 'pharmacological dissection'.[38]

The DSM was instrumental in these efforts, and companies turned to the DSM-III, with its 265 disorders, some of which did not have any pharmaceutical treatments attached to them, to see which might respond to their drug. The authors of the DSM sliced and diced disorders into discrete subtypes, accommodating pharmaceutical companies' needs, with anxiety being divided into panic disorder, phobic disorder, obsessive compulsive disorder, post-traumatic stress disorder, and generalised anxiety disorder.[39]

In the era of pharmaceutical dissection, each edition of the DSM has seen an increase in the number of mental diseases as well as the number of ways a mental illness can be diagnosed. The original DSM, published in 1952, had 106 forms of mental illness. DSM-II, in 1968, had 182. The radically biological DSM-III, in 1980, had 285. The fourth revision in 1994, had 307.[40] Today, the DSM contains almost 3 times the number of the first edition. These weren't new categories driven by the novel discoveries of a rapidly advancing science, either. As the DSM committee was devising its fifth edition, for example, the aim had initially been to work on the scientific basis underlying these diagnoses. The committee soon gave up; the evidence simply wasn't there.[41] Instead, they focused their efforts on creating more 'new' syndromes to be treated with yet more drug prescriptions. Despite the intermittent attempts to solidify the biological basis of the DSM, and with it, the profession of psychiatry, repeatedly, the only biology in sight was the impact drugs seemed to have on the brain, an impact that, we will see, makes much less sense biologically than it does economically.

With a growing untapped market of disorders to treat, SSRI companies threw themselves into a new form of innovation. They turned to the 'anxiety market', where tranquiliser drugs like Xanax had made their name.[42] SSRIs alleviated some of the symptoms of anxiety-associated depression, and this provided drug companies with all the justification they needed to take the step of marketing SSRIs as a treatment for a specific, as-yet unclaimed, form of anxiety in the DSM.

In 1999, the company, SmithKline Beecham secured a license from the FDA to sell its antidepressant Paxil for the DSM disorder of 'social phobia' or 'social anxiety disorder'. This wasn't a well-known disorder, so first they had to sell the disease. They launched a campaign, subtly titled: 'Imagine Being Allergic to People' and formed a patient advocacy group.[43] In December 2001, three months after the September 11 terrorist attacks, GlaxoSmithKline sent out its new commercials featuring distressed-looking people telling the camera: 'I'm always thinking something terrible is going to happen.' They reframed a very normal, reasonable response to a singular, seismic event, as a sign of illness. The diagnosis: generalised anxiety disorder. The solution: Paxil.[44]

In this sense, these drug companies were not just seizing on speculative diagnoses to make exaggerated claims for the benefits of their products for a range of symptoms that extended far beyond the modest improvements in a more limited range of symptoms they had actually observed (often, in animals, who hardly have comparable mental experiences to humans), they were also reframing, rather overtly, in their adverts, extreme events and traumatising experiences as individual problems with marketable solutions. As in the early days of Prozac, the solution was not to address the social system to mitigate stressful experiences or support people through them, but to medicate people to make them survive the inhumane conditions imposed on them.

Big pharma was becoming increasingly adept at powerfully and effectively convincing people that they *needed* drugs to heal themselves of a proliferating list of experiences reframed as brain-based disease. People didn't necessarily know that they were taking the same medication for a different disorder. And perhaps that wouldn't have mattered; many patients don't understand how the medication they take works. Only as the decade of the brain raged on, the opportunistic marketing strategies drew on this convenient narrative, and in doing so began to school the public in unproven scientific explanations that had significant consequences for the way patients understood themselves, and devastating consequences for the care they received.

The cost of failure

While the public continue to be bombarded with the serotonin imbalance explanation of depression, researchers today are becoming increasingly certain that all simplistic 'chemical imbalance' theories were probably wrong, and that no one understood how antidepressants worked.[45] This discrepancy between the state of research and public understanding persists to an extraordinary level. An extensive review published by two University College London psychiatrists in July 2022 made headlines[46] when it showed that there was still no clear evidence that serotonin levels or serotonin activity are responsible for depression. In their umbrella review of existing overviews of the evidence from each of the main areas of research into serotonin and depression, they showed that there is no accepted pharmacological mechanism for how antidepressants might affect depression.[47] This wasn't a new finding; the study was only comprehensively making a point that had been evident for some time. Yet despite a growing scepticism, half of all

SSRI patient leaflets continue to perpetuate the claim that these medicines help to correct certain chemical imbalances in the brain and that these are the symptoms of a brain-based illness.

That scientists don't understand exactly *how* SSRIs work does not in itself imply that antidepressants don't work; there are many people who, undeniably, have had their lives improved by taking these drugs, and, in any case, it is common practice in medicine to prescribe medication that is shown to be effective without understanding the underlying mechanism, from aspirin to morphine and penicillin. What is notable, however, is that an authoritative scientific narrative about how antidepressants work has persisted despite this widespread ignorance, and drug markets have relied on an inaccurate scientific narrative that has real, detrimental consequences for the way people and doctors understand the effects of antidepressants, and the extent to which they have (or haven't, in most cases) been able to explain why drug treatment often goes so wrong.

Again, maybe the untruths drug companies, enabled by governments, spread about the state of scientific knowledge could have been forgiven, if SSRIs were as safe and effective as the marketing campaigns made them out to be. But that soon turned out not to be the case. Whatever we make of the overall efficacy of antidepressants, it is undeniable that patients have been repeatedly and brutally confronted with the inaccuracy of the 'chemical imbalance' theory of depression through their experience of the disappointing and adverse effects of antidepressants on their wellbeing. This is evident in the numerous lawsuits these companies have faced over the past decades; a litany of allegations of suppressing information about side effects and causing patients life-inhibiting and life-ending harms. As early as the 1990s, Eli Lilly had been accused, in a series of lawsuits, of suppressing evidence that Prozac was capable of sparking violent or suicidal behaviour in patients who had never previously acted that way.[48] These drug companies have a history of repeatedly hiding and denying evidence of the harm their miracle drugs can do, making unsupported statements to patients that their drugs were safe, had no serious side effects and were easy to stop.

In 2023, BBC *Panorama* revealed how in 1996, Pfizer, originally the manufacturer of sertraline (today the UK's most common antidepressant) attempted to conceal the possible withdrawal effects of its SSRI. A confidential memo revealed how employees discussed how the drug company would suppress information to regulators in Norway: 'We should not volunteer to describe the withdrawal symptoms, but have an agreed list prepared in case they insist,' the memo read.[49] Some of the withdrawal reactions the memo refers to include sensory disturbances, sweating, nausea, insomnia, tremors, agitation and anxiety.

In 2008, Dr Erick Turner, working as a reviewer at the US's Food and Drug Administration (FDA), conducted a study that showed that companies were publishing clinical trials very selectively.[50] He compared the trials published in the literature to those registered by the FDA, and found that the negative trials, where the drug did not outperform the placebo, were not being reported. This is how drug companies gave the impression that pills worked most of the time, when in reality, almost half the studies were negative. This allowed companies to report, and psychiatrists to believe that whatever the side effects, the cost-benefit ratio for SSRIs was overall positive. Side effects and devastating withdrawal symptoms may have been worth it, had the drugs worked most of the time.

As SSRIs continued to flow, unobstructed by inconvenient findings, from bench to bedside, patients increasingly reported severe symptoms when they tried to come off SSRIs. Often, they described their symptoms coming off the drug as worse than the initial symptoms of their depression. One recurring experience was that of sexual numbing, today known as post-SSRI sexual dysfunction (PSSD), and described by sufferers as chemical castration,[51] which involves an experience of persistent changes in sexual function for an extended period after stopping SSRIs. Repeatedly, these reports were ignored. Online forums allowed patients to connect, and eventually led a psychologist with first-hand experience of PSSD to publish an academic paper that gave legitimacy to the diagnosis.[52] The Royal College of Psychiatrists did not officially recognise withdrawal symptoms as a serious concern until 2019, when it finally published updated information on withdrawal. Until then, guidance used by the NHS and the College continued to assert that withdrawal was mostly mild and short-lived – lasting no more than about a week. In a 2023 BBC *Panorama* documentary, Professor Wendy Burn, who was the College's president at the time, reluctantly apologised for this longstanding dismissal of patients' repeatedly reported experience.

Despite the ongoing controversy about the benefit-risk ratio of SSRIs, today, at the very least, it is known that SSRIs are not the quick fix they were purported to be in the decade of the brain. A comprehensive study from the University of Oxford suggests antidepressants do help some people, at least in the short-term, but only work 15 per cent better than placebos.[53] On average, the benefits are relatively modest, and the way people respond varies, with some not responding at all – a far cry from the miracle cure they are marketed as.

All this is not to say that for those who benefit from antidepressants, they are not a life-saving intervention. For those whose distress has pushed them to a ledge, and are struggling to keep on living, let alone undergo therapy, 15 per cent could make all the difference. For some who take antidepressants intermittently when they feel themselves sinking, it is also helpful to understand their disorder as a chemical imbalance, one where, from time to time, they need a top-up. This may give them a sense of control over what might feel like a frightening and inexplicable change in their experience. This view might help clarify their needs and distance them from a mechanism that they may otherwise experience as a personal failing. Yet, for those whose distress can't be managed so straightforwardly, this explanation might exacerbate feelings of hopelessness, and reinforce feelings that they are broken, when not even these drugs, supposedly based on a mechanistic understanding of the chemicals in the brain, work on them. This is especially evident in the accounts of the people who experienced withdrawal symptoms as they were coming off antidepressants, which, given that these weren't even recognised by the psychiatric institution, were mistaken for signs of relapse. This led people to believe that they were dependent on artificial chemicals, held together only by drugs, when in reality, the chemicals were actually causing their withdrawal symptoms. There are also the people for whom antidepressants make no difference, who need to unpack the cause of their depression in their life histories or current situation. These people need a different language that shows them that their distress isn't their fault and doesn't define them. To these people, the explanation that mental distress is the product of a set of social and cultural conditions, will likely prove more helpful. For these people, and they do seem to be the majority, we need to find better metaphors and better systems to support them.

Today, it is largely recognised that antidepressants are not a one-size-fits-all cure, and definitely not the personality boosters they were considered to be in their heyday. Yet the pharmaceutical view of depression lives on. In the media, drugs continue to represent the cutting edge of science and the horizon of hope for mental health. We may as a culture have become sceptical about the hope of SSRIs, but several decades' worth of fervent marketing has left an indelible imprint on our thinking. While we understand that drugs are not the one-stop cures we thought they were, all the discussions and treatments we see are still very much rooted in an understanding of diagnoses like depression as problems with the brain. This biological view assumes that mental disease can be definitively, medically, known and cured, and it remains the party line in a world in which there is little leeway for individual adjustment, where people are expected to adapt to the demands of society, rather than having their individual needs met. A drug to keep up with the demands of work is still, for many, the closest they'll get to feeling good, or least like a functioning member of society. Our lifeline depends on the belief that our distress is generic and can be treated generically; that our problem exists in the exact same formation as everyone else's, in the brain.

Brainy solutions

The plan announced by the NIH in 2005 was to create an environment for innovation. And they did just that. Besides the boom in drug sales, the field of neuroscience more generally has been equally lucrative. While growth rates are slowing, the market value continues to grow nonetheless. The global neuroscience market is currently worth around $612 billion and is predicted to grow to $720.8 billion by 2026.[54] The hope of a steady flow of research to fuel innovation has equally become manifest, with two decades of prolific research behind us. And yet, in the hyper-paced, streamlined flow between research and industry, the quality of research, and quality of clinical outcomes, has yet to benefit from this innovation landscape. The hope and promise of health on which the entire trajectory from research to industry was predicated remains an ever-receding horizon.

That is partly because the translational landscape fosters innovation, not better care for patients. The push to transform research into products has put researchers under immense pressure. With universities more closely tied to industry, researchers have been subjected to market laws, where competition is ever greater to produce robust and applicable findings that can be translated into clinical applications. Researchers race to publish high quantities of research quickly, and in the 'high impact' journals that only print the most novel or news-worthy findings: generally, those with prospects for commercialisation.

This rat-race has led researchers increasingly to misrepresent data.[55] Pressure to publish cutting-edge results also disincentivises replication studies that are necessary to confirm and validate findings. This is, of course, essential, especially if the goal is to apply insights in a clinical setting with real human patients. Yet the British Neuroscience Association have recognised that in the current translational climate, scientific knowledge is vulnerable to a bias that 'skews scientific understanding, contributes to hyped expectations, and jeopardises the translation of research to real-world applications.'[56] Some have even begun to refer to a crisis of reproducibility in neuroscience.[57]

While the pipeline undoubtedly achieved its aims of maximising profits, it is doubtful that this widely lauded hotbed for innovation actually benefits science. Many scientists themselves have argued that the culture of fierce competition for funding, high-profile publications, and the recognition of colleagues has undermined the values of scientific practice. Research, they say, is rewarded for flash rather than substance. This is particularly true in the field of neuroimaging. This technology that allows scientists to look directly into the brain has been a key area of translational hope and investment. It was hoped that this technology would be used, not just to identify the effects of stroke and brain injury, or supporting surgery with brain maps, but also for finding abnormalities connected to the DSM disorders. The field was shaken by a 2016 announcement that the rate of false positives in functional imaging could be much higher than expected due to inadequate statistical control,[58] and this was not the first finding of this kind.[59]

The findings in neuroimaging have fallen well short of expectations. A 2016 analysis of over 500 functional MRI (fMRI)[60] studies of psychiatric patients (around 20,000 people) failed to find any differential brain activations corresponding to specific disorders as defined by the DSM; in other words, this type of brain imaging technology may have allowed a window onto the brain, but it did not reveal the brain disease psychiatrists had hoped to find.[61] Scientists in the area of neuroimaging have learned a great deal about the functioning of different areas of the brain, have identified specific genes involved in brain development, and better understand how brain pathways are mediated by neurotransmitters and proteins.[62] None of these advances, though, have described or identified the mental disorders in the DSM as purely the function of brain activity. The hope that psychiatry would be a profession concerned with identifying and treating brain diseases hasn't materialised. And, because this brain-based treatment has been its sole focus, neither has its ability to better support people. In 2018, the American Psychiatrist Association (APA) published a position paper stating 'neuroimaging has yet to have a significant impact on the diagnosis or treatment of individual patients in clinical settings.'[63]

In 2010, Tom Insel, the director of the National Institute of Mental Health in the US, even announced that the hunt for biological mechanisms underlying DSM categories had failed. The project hadn't worked and, not just that, there had been no 'marked increase in the rate of recovery from mental illness, nor a detectable decrease in suicide or homelessness – each of which is associated with a failure to recover from mental illness.'[64] His solution? More neuroscience.

The hype and hope around brain science for psychiatry created an environment conducive to profit, based on unrealistic promises and flimsy findings. Yet it also didn't allow for the benefits that neuroscience's products might bring as tools, rather than cures. The overblown hope of a generic cure for all humanity's ills misses the more tempered understanding of the context-dependent value that neuroscientific diagnostics, medicine and technologies might bring in clinical practice. Neuroimaging could, for example, be used to identify those experiences that *do* have a biological component. Infection, toxicity, inflammation, gut–brain dysregulation and traumatic brain injury can all induce experiences which according to the DSM might otherwise be diagnosed as a psychiatric disorder.[65] These phenomena can be investigated in their own right, and the symptoms associated with them could potentially be targeted. But these biological mechanisms have to be distinguished from psychiatric diagnoses. In fact, if anything, they should be used to parse apart psychiatry from neuroscience 'proper' – to reinforce a separation between the specific mechanisms that can be understood using biological tools, and the mental experiences that will always require other ways of knowing. We will see how, once we delve into the social causes of mental distress, psychiatric interventions, including drugs, start to look increasingly like tools, rather than cures, that need to be used as part of a much more holistic effort to help people face the multifaceted challenges that cause them to suffer. From this perspective, the idea that a drug could ever have solved issues of housing stress or fear of violence as an issue that exists only in the brain looks absurd. The brain might register the impact of these experiences, but brain mechanisms may not be where we look to help someone with them. The pipeline view obfuscates this broader perspective, and the (less profitable) solutions it may bring.

Pipeline dreams

In the context of the underwhelming outcome of neuroscientific applications, we can begin to see how the story of SSRIs is much more than an argument for better government regulation over drug markets (although this is also crucial). We need to question the pipeline view of mental health itself that continues to tie a brain-based view to the need for medical solutions. This view sees mental disease as a problem that exists in the brain, individuals as passive consumers, rather than people with individual needs, and mental struggle as a biological problem to be fixed, rather than symptoms of not just individual, but social problems.

The hype and hope around neuroscientific and medical cures for psychiatric conditions is reinforced in culture at large. Brain breakthroughs in psychiatry continue to receive disproportionate media attention. We see this, not least, in an ever-burgeoning genre of books that straddles the line of neuroscience and self-help – bestsellers like psychiatrist Bessel van der Kolk's *The Body Keeps the Score*, *What Happened to You? Conversations on Trauma, Resilience, and Healing*, a collab between psychiatrist Bruce D. Perry and Oprah Winfrey, or clinical psychologist Lisa Feldman Barrett's *How Emotions Are Made: The Secret Life of the Brain*. These books offer brain-based theories (many disproven or, at best, as-yet-unproven) for our emotions and behaviour, along with the promise of 'life-hacks', ways to manage our human distress.

It isn't hard to see why these books resonate with so many; they appeal to that same biological hope we have seen – the hope of an end to our suffering, in a world that offers us only biological explanations and solutions. Brain scans feature heavily. The fMRI scan, now over thirty years old, is repeatedly presented as the brain's reliable translator. This is despite the many challenges to its reliability, let alone questions about what brain scans really tell us. One of my favourite scientific critiques involved putting a dead salmon through an fMRI.[66] The tongue-in-cheek experiment revealed detected activity in the fish's dead brain, proving how easily false positives can be wrangled from brain scan findings, and proving to anyone who looked to brain scans for straightforward maps of brain activity that this is far from the window onto human consciousness we imagined. The books consumed by large swathes of the population in the hope of some reprieve to their suffering, report much outdated and unfounded science, and greatly overstate its findings, fuelling that biological hope of its eager readers who lack the scientific literacy to critique the findings they are presented with.

These books also fuel the translational pipeline, as scientists, whose funding streams rely increasingly on popular support (reflected in the decisions of funding bodies), keep the biological hope alive. At best, they oversimplify and overstate the takeaways of neuroscientific research; at worst, they rehash neuroscientific ideas that are already outmoded.[67] They rely on theories that gain traction on social media, catchy terms that rely on reductive quasi-scientific narratives in a society primed to find comfort in the prospect of scientific advancement. 'Mirror neurons', for example, are widely referred to as a supposed biological mechanism for the capacity for empathy. When monkeys watch other monkeys eating a banana, the explanation goes, some of the same neurons are activated for the observer as the observed. While these neurons have not been identified in humans, the theory has travelled through popularisations of the science as established fact.[68] 'Lizard brains' are another favourite – the idea that humans have a primitive brain centre that acts on instinct – long debunked but remarkably persistent.[69] These theories all reaffirm the inevitability and certainty of human emotion and suffering as brain-based. All the while, of course, directing our gazes from the social systems that can foster empathy, as well as distress.

Humane translations

None of this is to deny the relief drugs or medical treatment might bring patients struggling right now. But, again, the question when it comes to neuroscientific breakthroughs is not just whether the drugs work, but also, crucially: *What are we missing?* What are we not investigating when we allow research to be driven by financial flows? What opportunities for improving health and preventing harm are we foregoing when we prioritise neuroscientific studies and treatment? Animated by the widespread societal and political faith placed in biomedical innovations, the translational flow is stronger than ever. To change the approach, and improve the efficacy of responses to mental health, we will need to regulate and reshape that pipeline.

Because, as ever, medical myopia affects those already socioeconomically disadvantaged in our society the most. People with lower socioeconomic status, also the group who are most likely to experience mental distress, are more likely to receive medication, rather than therapy in comparison to people from higher-income backgrounds.[70] They are more likely to be funnelled down the pipeline of market-driven medical and medicalised therapies and more likely to experience the associated neglect of the underlying cause of their distress. They will not have the option of supplementing their drugs with more extensive, self-funded, therapy, for example. They are more likely to find themselves on waiting lists for government-funded support.[71] Black British people, too, are about 4 times more likely than White people to be given psychoactive medication than talking therapy.[72] The same is true for all ethnic minorities compared to whites in the US.[73] Whatever we are told about the promise of psychiatric science today, unacknowledged classist, racist and sexist views are driving (predominantly middle-class and White) doctors' decisions on the treatment, rather than scientific evidence.

When help finally comes for these people, their distress may have driven them to other, distressing (conscious and unconscious) coping mechanisms, like self-harm, or psychosis. In the current system, these issues are less likely to be met with the compassion of the therapist than the hand of the law; and, of course, this is especially true where race intersects with class: 7.7 per cent of prisoners in England and Wales are Black, although Black people only make up 4.4 per cent of the population,[74] and in the US, Black Americans are incarcerated in state prisons at nearly 5 times the rate of white Americans. Once incarcerated, prison has a proven track record of fostering addiction and violence.

Once released, with a criminal record, they will be less likely to find employment, to lose their homes, and so their jobs, as they are swept up by the social drift that pulls them deeper into poverty and despair. The social ramifications of disparities in care are monumental. As ever, flows of capital are impersonal and favour the mental wellbeing of no one, but, in combination with the prejudices and structural inequality built into medical systems and internalised by medical professionals, the medical model particularly fails to meet the needs of people who are struggling with the real social and psychological problems that stem from poverty. In today's political and economic climate, financial flows imbue specific kinds of knowledge with the mark of 'potential', 'progress', 'hope' – and authority. Medicine, pharmaceuticals and brain science are the order of the day. But by thinking in terms of medical and medical-model solutions, by prioritising these above others, we neglect the resources and support services that are most crucial to the people who are least able to benefit from the spoils of profits from the miracle cures we are constantly being sold. This is how most people are actually harmed by them.

The pipeline cure precludes the possibility of finding other, perhaps better, forms of support for people. The diagnostic model in psychiatry frames mental experiences as generically knowable and curable, and then promises universal cures. But, as the discussion of people's social environments already shows, this misses the complex and multi-factorial causes of suffering, as well as people's highly variable and individual needs. Besides the assumption that profits must equate to progress, the belief in the translational pipeline's potential to cure mental illness also depends on the assumption that a generic cure for psychiatric disease is possible; that the value of these products can be carried from the lab to the clinic and applied to any human being, to achieve similar results. The pipeline does not slow to incorporate people's priorities; as we have seen, drug companies have even *created* markets, generated a demand, rather than responding to real needs.

One way to redirect the flow of translation towards people's actual needs, is to involve them in the priority setting, bring together patients, carers and clinicians to work together to agree on key future areas of research. The James Lind Alliance,[75] for example, is a non-profit organisation that facilitates priority setting partnerships of this kind. The priorities that are set through these discussions often challenge preconceptions held by the research community about what is important to patients. In contrast to the emphasis on finding cures in the translational research pipeline, what emerged in the studies on Parkinson's disease, for example, is that patients are more concerned with improving quality of life through earlier diagnosis or better management of distressing symptoms. Indeed, this is a recurring finding across other areas in neuroscience. Patient and public involvement that paired researchers with people living with dementia has also shown that maintaining a higher level of independence, or delaying disease progression, are often more important to patients than the development of treatments or cures.[76]

The evidence collected from these discussions can be used to justify funding of research areas focused on these social and psychological areas, as well as medical tools or (where appropriate) cures that might otherwise go neglected. Studies like these can be used to draw attention to the developments that would inspire the most hope in patients, rather than economic stakeholders, and present the possibility, working within a system that connects evidence to clinical applications, to draw on a different knowledge base to the studies on the physical mechanisms of the brain. Of course, the extent to which these insights will be implemented, will depend on governance and policy, and on where we, as a society, place our hope for our mental wellbeing: in medical hype, or in real, lived, experience. And, we'll see, for psychiatry itself to play its role in putting people's experience at the centre of mental healthcare, will require overhaul of the power dynamics that have long been its structuring principle.

3

The Myth of Personality Disorders: BPD

Personality disorders are different from other psychiatric disorders. While they are included in the DSM in the same medical paradigm, they are generally considered by psychiatrists as intractable compared to the other mental disorders. 'Personality', after all, refers to a characteristic way of behaving, experiencing life, and of perceiving and interpreting oneself, other people, events and situations. For people with personality disorders, these patterns of behaviour, cognition and inner experience are 'disturbed' in such a way that they cause problems in interpersonal functioning or their relationship with themselves.[1] In the DSM, personality disorders are separated into 'clusters': Cluster A, containing disorders described by 'odd or eccentric' behaviour, such as paranoid personality disorder, Cluster B, containing 'dramatic, emotional, or erratic' disorders, which includes both BPD and HPD or narcissistic personality disorder, and Cluster C, containing 'anxious or fearful' disorders, like OCD.[2]

The language used to cluster these disorders based on descriptive similarities betrays the judgements that diagnosis of a personality disorder necessitates; 'odd', 'eccentric' or 'dramatic'. Whatever the standardised tools used to assess individuals, these descriptions will be made by people holding unconscious and conscious cultural beliefs about what constitutes a norm. The International Classification of Diseases (ICD), the psychiatric manual maintained by the World Health Organisation and more commonly used outside the US, acknowledges the connection between personality disorders and 'personal and social disruption',[3] so there is some reference to the potential causes of a disruption in the personality, which also suggests the experience is not inherent to the person. Nonetheless, like the DSM, the ICD still marks these disorders as distinct from other mental health conditions.

In both manuals, other conditions, such as mood disorders or psychotic disorders, are considered more episodic and characterised by a distinct onset of symptoms. They differ from the personality disorders which are presented as incalcitrant, rooted in that most unchanging aspect of ourself.

While all personality disorders have a reputation for being intractable, borderline personality disorder (BPD),[4] also known as emotionally unstable personality disorder (EUPD), has, more than many of the other personality disorders, long been linked to patients deemed 'difficult'. When compared to the other 'emotional' or 'erratic' Cluster B personality disorders, BPD stands out as a confusing amalgam of them all. It sits somewhere between the heights of psychopathy expressed in ASPD, or the harmless exhibitionism of HPD, as something in between; both emotional and aggressive, invoking fear and dismissal. It absorbs qualities of all into a muddled image of a case that is difficult to define, and so, in the psychiatric method, also difficult to treat.

According to the 2013 fifth edition of the DSM, the essential feature of BPD is a pervasive pattern of instability of self-image, interpersonal relationships, and emotions that begins by early adulthood and is present in a variety of contexts. To be diagnosed, an individual must either have an unstable self-image or unstable goals, must be inordinately sensitive or have unstable personal relationships, and show what are deemed to be pathological degrees of mood changes or anxiety, fear of abandonment, low moods, impulsivity, risk-taking, and hostility.[5] It is associated with significant psychiatric mortality and morbidity; approximately 10 per cent of individuals diagnosed with BPD will eventually take their lives,[6] and people with BPD are still, in many mental healthcare settings, considered untreatable.

From its origins, borderline personality disorder, BPD, has offered a blurry zone, used to mark people who were deemed to be less than sane, but not quite mad. As a murky, poorly defined place, it has also lent itself to underinformed judgements. It easily became a way to mark people who were deemed resistant to treatment intended for the regularly 'neurotic', but unsuitable for the treatment designed for the properly mad. Many critics have claimed the category reflects clinicians' own unease or impatience more than it does the problems of the client. It is a bracket of patients, they claim, that registers the limits of the profession. And it is true that, since the early origins of BPD, we can see how the theories underpinning the diagnosis have reflected pejorative judgement, more than helpful science.

The basis for BPD was developed by the Austrian-born American psychoanalyst Otto Kernberg in the 1970s. The concept had existed for over a century, under different names, as a liminal zone somewhere between sanity and full-fledged madness. These patients were often considered too well for the hospital but too ill for the couch

– a dead-end kind of diagnosis. Kernberg gave some definition to the concept by rooting this 'borderline' in the personality. He was convinced that his patients at New York Presbyterian Hospital weren't just experiencing borderline states of madness, but that their personality was organised entirely differently, and that their condition was inherited. He introduced borderline personality organisation (BPO) in 1975[7] as a 'level' of personality organisation that was distinct from psychotic personality organisation, where a sense of reality is completely gone, and distinct from neurotic personality organisation, where, unlike BPO, which was characterised by a weakened sense of self, the self remained intact.[8]

BPO was a broad umbrella term, a catch-all that included patients with anorexia, bulimia, and other severe personality disorders, such as hypomanic, schizotypal, antisocial, psychopathic, paranoid and narcissistic. Kernberg also used BPO to describe patients who had been diagnosed with the new label of 'histrionic personality' characterised with those 'hysteric' traits (dramatic emotional, seductive, suggestible), and whose 'interpersonal functioning' was also highly unstable.[9] BPO, which would become BPD in 1980, was a form of hysteria, but amplified by a degree of instability that was somehow more threatening than hysteria alone.

And so, an ill-defined wastebasket of psychiatry for cases that seemed to fall outside agreed-upon diagnoses became a personality disorder.

In Kernberg's decision to frame the traits of people deemed somehow abnormal, but not necessarily insane, as a personality disorder, he laid the foundations for a remarkably flexible category for marking all kinds of non-conformity. A diagnosis with a personality disorder today, according to the DSM, means that 'one's way of thinking, feeling and behaving deviates from the expectations of the culture, causes distress or problems functioning, and lasts over time.'[10] This mention of culture is incredibly revealing, because it shows us how easily nonconformity could be diagnosed as a disorder. If the dominant culture is sexist, heteronormative, racist or ableist, and psychiatrists' ideas about what constitutes 'normality' are shaped by that dominant culture, a personality quickly becomes disordered when it deviates from a stereotype, or when it upholds a stereotype that is generally pathologised (like being feminine, or, historically, and in many places still, being gay).

Since Kernberg's blueprint, BPD has been framed as an aspect of a person's deep-rooted personality, rather than a set of physical, psychological or emotional symptoms triggered by, for example, trauma. But it isn't really clear why. In Kernberg's definition of BPO, for example, he lists criteria like 'identity sense' or 'reality testing' or 'anxiety',[11] which are aspects of mental experience that could just as well be affected by environmental factors, like stressful experiences, and biological factors, like hormonal changes, or genetic disposition, just as the other mental health conditions, like psychosis or depression.

Today, in the high-tech scientific era, the framing of BPD as a problem in the person has guided research in a very particular direction. There exists a whole plethora of studies on the genetics of BPD, presenting the argument that the disorder is not only inherent but also inherited; neither of which, of course, have been proven. It would be difficult to prove, considering that, as we have seen, it isn't entirely clear what the diagnosis actually describes; many of the criteria associated with the disorder are clustered symptoms, like anxiety, anger or depression, which could be easily understood as reactions to a situation rather than personality traits. Since it isn't clear whether BPD exists in the form it is currently described, it is difficult to imagine how this undefined diagnosis could even be inherited. Moreover, even if specific genes were linked to the susceptibility in a person, this does not make the need to understand the impact of traumatic experiences any less pressing: these genes need to be activated or deactivated, and that happens based on environmental factors, like trauma. Claims about the innate, genetic existence of the disease are misleading but also forcefully distract from the events and experiences that may have brought on certain reactions, and that may need legal, or societal action and change. The diagnosis of BPD, in this light, functions more as a barometer for social disruption than a measure of mental functioning.

Most importantly, rooting problems in personalities, rather than experiences, affects the treatment available. The view that the symptoms associated with disorders like BPD are personality problems can easily lead to a stigmatising view of the individual as inherently dysfunctional.[12] When the perception is that these disorders are lodged firmly in a person, rather than triggered by environmental or biological events, psychiatrists might be less optimistic about the treatment they can offer.[13] In fact, if psychiatrists consider mental disorders their domain of expertise, defining personality disorders as a slightly different category means that some psychiatrists consider these outside their purview. Ultimately, whether someone is diagnosed with a personality disorder, or another mental health disorder, will determine whether they can access psychiatric treatment, like long-term therapy or medication. For people who need some kind of support or a lifeline, a BPD diagnosis might paradoxically bar them from getting the help they need. And so, the personality disorder easily becomes a category used to demarcate people as they were in Kernberg's time and before, as somehow not quite normal, but also, now not deserving of the proper treatment afforded to someone who is deemed legitimately unwell, and not just branded as 'difficult'.

A female disease?

Whereas hysterical women were considered 'damaged', BPD women are considered 'difficult', and even 'dangerous'.[14]

Like hysteria, BPD is diagnosed not only but mainly in women, and mainly in women who have experienced sexual abuse. Since the late 1970s, scientists and feminists alike have been building an evidence base for the relationship between BPD and sexual abuse. These studies showed that histories of childhood physical and sexual abuse are common in those diagnosed with BPD, and sexual abuse is consistently and significantly reported more often by those diagnosed with BPD than by those diagnosed with depression or other personality disorders.[15] Childhood sexual abuse is also less common in samples of people with milder or fewer BPD traits or symptoms.[16] Studies show that 81 per cent of patients diagnosed with BPD had reported experiences of child abuse, of which 71 per cent reported physical abuse, 68 per cent sexual abuse, and 62 per cent witnessing serious domestic violence.[17] This is compared to 17–45 per cent in control groups that include people not diagnosed with BPD, sometimes with other mental health disorders.[18]

Viewed through the lens of trauma, however, many of the symptoms associated with BPD, like mistrust or anger, seem less pathological and more like necessary coping strategies in threatening contexts. These aren't the symptoms of a disease, but of a healthy coping mechanism. How useful it is, then, to pathologise the very emotions that may be essential to defending yourself in the face of abuse?

Anger, for example, is an emotion used to assert boundaries. It is a claiming of space, or a demand for recognition, both from yourself and others. Anger is importantly unleashed in the face of injustice. When a person feels they are not being respected, when they feel their boundaries are being transgressed, their freedoms infringed upon, anger is expressed. To pathologise this response in people who have experienced trauma is not to give them a diagnosis that enables a cure, but to deny them the agency to protect and defend themselves. BPD, in this way, also drives to a head a perception that exists across mental health systems, that patients are 'risky,' potentially pose harm to themselves and others, and so need to be controlled. This view is widespread among psychiatrists and policymakers who when designing care systems, prioritise 'risk management' – not just in the criminal justice system, where psychiatrists' assessments have a weighty impact on sentencing, parole or early release, but across all mental health services, where risk assessments conducted by psychiatrists can determine whether people will be sectioned, or involuntarily treated or contained. This policing function is an accepted part of psychiatrists' jobs.[19]

This general orientation around risk across psychiatry means that, rather than working with the causes for behaviour perceived as angry or aggressive, which often involve trauma, the response becomes punitive: to restrain, tranquilise, or generally stop people from behaving a certain way. While in rare cases, this may be necessary, this assumption that the patient poses a danger to themselves and others precludes the possibility, usually very present, that a person can be supported in making their own choices about their own care. A more empowering approach would start with a more compassionate view that takes into account the circumstances that make people behave a certain way.

Borderline personality disorder describes a special place reserved predominantly for women who have experienced sexual trauma. But that isn't explicit in its psychiatric definition. Instead, their behaviours are framed as pathological and stemming from a disordered personality. This widespread misrepresentation of primarily women's experiences mirrors the mechanisms we have seen with hysteria. This sleight of hand has been made possible by a history of institutions conspiring to place the causes of sexual violence against women in their wombs, neurology or personalities. Today, almost half of the women who qualify for a histrionic or a borderline diagnosis meet the criteria for both disorders.[20] In light of their link to sexual trauma, BPD and hysteria start to look like two sides of a coin, connected to two stereotypes of damaged and dangerous women.

Clare Shaw is a writer and campaigner who was diagnosed with BPD in her early twenties. When we spoke in 2023, Shaw told me how she was first admitted to a psychiatric ward after overdosing, but how she had already had a history of self-harming extending back to age ten that had gone unacknowledged by her family or medical professionals. She described her presenting symptoms at the time in medical terms: suicidal and self-harming behaviours, intense moods, chronic feelings of emptiness, despair, an eating disorder. These, she believes, led to her diagnosis. Yet distress in response to difficulties in relationships, seen in context, are not unreasonable responses.

Shaw also cited the fact that she didn't respond to antidepressants, and that she asked questions, so that she was probably perceived as a less compliant – and therefore 'difficult' – patient. She is queer, which was equally treated as problematic, as transgressing the expectations of femininity expected of her. Being diagnosed with BPD, she said, reinforced the feelings she'd already had around her family, of her being the problem, of her personality being at fault, of being born manipulative, a liar, bad, too clever and difficult. The way she was treated by clinicians further reinforced this disdain. She was judged, dismissed, and physically restrained and contained. All the while, the reasons for the regime of 'care' were kept from her. She only became aware of her diagnosis when she caught sight of paperwork several years later – she hadn't even been informed.

Nor had anyone acknowledged the real source of her suffering: that she had grown up in a context of sexual abuse, physical violence and alcoholism. Suffice to say, medical treatment was not helpful for Shaw. Yet the misdirected and often outright harmful treatment she experienced wasn't even the real crux of the problem for her; rather, what haunts her to this day are the long-term detrimental consequences the language of diagnosis has had for her sense of self, as well as the long-unacknowledged trauma.

Shaw told me about the impact that the language of 'disorder' had on her: 'Services are years behind me now and I live with having been constructed as a disordered person, and I live with what that's done to my sense of myself. And it's a conscious daily effort to reframe my more difficult parts and experiences and not to view them as signs of a disordered personality. If we tell people that their feelings, their ways of coping are disordered, it will have lasting effects.' From this perspective, we can start to imagine what better support for people currently diagnosed with BPD might look like. Rather than diagnosing someone with BPD, it might be more important to look to the problems in their lived environment, and to help them find a safe place to live first. It might then be more useful to help individuals make sense of their own behaviour as coping mechanisms, and to work with them to understand how their past and present made these strategies necessary. It will eventually be much more helpful to support people to find their own alternative coping mechanisms that might better serve them, always in light of what feels possible and safe to them. This kind of response, of course, would require more than psychiatry, but a coordinated response involving a range of social workers, psychotherapists, local communities and perhaps psychiatrists. This kind of response can only emerge from a view of mental distress that isn't primarily a personality problem. It would require us to move beyond a pathologising view of behaviour, towards one of people trying their best in problematic conditions.

The double-bind

Shaw isn't the first to point to how diagnoses like BPD are used to punish non-conforming behaviour. Second-wave feminists, for example, did a lot to reveal how hysteria worked to shore up female gender roles at a time of social transition. Betty Friedman famously made the argument in her 1963 manifesto, *The Feminine Mystique*, that what had been called a hysterical neurosis of housewives throughout 1950s America was actually a normal response to the conditions of being trapped, bored and alone. Women found that they weren't alone in their experience, and as they did so, they named the problem they were facing. What Friedman had called 'the problem with no name' wasn't hysteria, or any other diagnosis that punishes behaviours that, in context, are entirely reasonable. The 'problem with no name' was, in fact, oppression itself.

With a newfound language, women began to form consciousness-raising groups where they made sense of their own experience, located the source of their discontent in the world they existed in, rather than their own repressed 'feminine' sexuality. As they found connection and solidarity, they started to push for social solutions for what had always been presented to them as individual, internal defects for which women themselves were to blame. They started to push for social support, for societal rights, for sexual freedom. Through this combination of community and an understanding of the social forces that limited them, women found themselves suddenly feeling a lot better, having relieved themselves of the societal gaslighting that made society's problems their problem.

The persistence of hysteria, second-wave feminists went on to argue over the following decades, was not a disease that had persisted through time; its recalcitrance only proved one thing: the doggedness of a patriarchal method. Hysteria was a fluid term but an even more malleable method that had, for centuries, recommended 'cures' for women that always involved subjugation. The recommended treatment, according to Freud's theory of psychoanalysis, had remained what it had been for centuries: marrying and having babies, only now it was in order to regain the 'lost' phallus.[21] But Freud had also added something new, and insidious, into the mix – that new theory, told via a seductive story that became the basis for a system of understanding identity and subjectivity to this day. In the Oedipal story, women are always constituted as the negated obverse of men – the castrated 'other' left behind in the man's completion of the Oedipal process, the woman whose lack of a penis condemns her to spend her life looking to fill that void 'normally' by committing herself to motherhood. Women could overcome the guilt and shame Freud believed them to feel about their sexual desires by integrating this with a 'healthy' maternal identity. The basis of Freudian psychoanalysis, the 'invention' of modern hysteria, in this sense, is also the affirmation in modern medicine of women's necessary function as bearers of children.

Freud's theories became useful patriarchal stories. When Betty Friedman drew attention to the plight of American women, she did so by showing how Freud's psychoanalysis had been used in the 1950s to rationalise the social movement ushering women back into the home in post war America. Freud had become what she called an 'American ideology' that turned women's understandable reaction to the drudgery of an under-stimulating existence into an illness. These women felt alone, isolated in their respective households, the private sphere in which their lives and also their sorrows were contained. Freud's emphasis on individual therapy aligned well with this social fragmentation and placed the onus of responsibility on the individual to rectify their deviation.

Displays of emotion, of any kind, are likely to discredit any person in the eyes of a society structured along gendered binaries. In the case of BPD, though, this leads to an overemphasis in diagnosis on the emotionality over the substance of a person's words; emotionality is now what needs to be treated, not any assault or abuse that necessitated such a response in the first place.[22] A societal preoccupation with reason and 'rationality', associated with the mind, has also long situated women on the side of irrationality, as well as a set of other gendered binaries, emotion, nature and the body, in opposition to the male reason, discourse, culture and mind.[23] In a world where for a woman to be well is to be feminine, and to be feminine is to be always dysfunctional, there is no way out – there is no 'recovery'. Despite the efforts of second-wave feminists to expose hysteria as social control parading as diagnosis, and despite their attempts to show that the problem was societal, not medical, psychiatry only doubled down with its narrow diagnoses, now also backed by an emerging pharmaceutical industry that continued to sedate America's dissatisfied women.

BPD further reinforced hysteria's double bind, where women are pathologised both for conforming to, and for failing to conform to, expectations of feminine passivity.[24] In the case of BPD, the diagnosis could be applied to women who fail to live up to their gender role because they expressed anger and aggression. But it could equally be diagnosed in women who conformed 'too strongly' to feminine ideals, by internalising anger and expressing this through self-destructive behaviour, like self-harm or suicide.[25] In this double bind, emotions regarded as too feminine or unfeminine are pathologised in the same way.

The psychiatric response to 'borderline symptoms' can be seen as an extension of this cultural mechanism that inhibits a person's chance of advocating for themselves, let alone participating in public life. And it isn't just women. Though today, still, around 75 per cent of people diagnosed with BPD are women,[26] BPD is also more likely to be diagnosed in queer people when they present with the same symptoms as a heterosexual person, who is more likely to be diagnosed with an anxiety disorder.[27] This reflects a psychiatric judgement of whose emotions are appropriate with reference to their conception of a 'norm'. This is how normal emotional responses, like anger or a fear of abandonment following a traumatic loss, can be – and frequently are – judged to be inappropriate, while any reasonable causes for these emotions are not investigated. This, of course, has implications for women, but men too, who will be subjected to the same denigration if they show what are perceived as 'feminine', and so 'inferior', emotionality.

A question of care

It is now widely recognised that many women with a diagnosis of BPD have a history of trauma, and although this is backed up with data, this has not translated into more appropriate treatment in mainstream care.[28] In light of the consistent findings of the link between BPD and abuse, some have tried to reframe BPD itself as a complex form of post-traumatic stress disorder.[29]

While in Europe and the UK there have been moves to include a version of complex PTSD in the ICD-11,[30] in North America, there are still no plans to include complex PTSD in the DSM. This lack of formal recognition also makes scientists internationally reluctant to dedicate their careers to exploring an approach to psychological distress that roots its cause in trauma. The dearth of funding means that there is a limited evidence base on complex PTSD, or on the most effective treatments, which further serves to discredit this perspective that legitimises the trauma view of the symptoms currently associated with BPD. The DSM is also key to insurance coverage, special services in schools, disability benefits and treatments. As long as complex PTSD does not officially exist, medical insurance companies will not reimburse sufferers for psychological treatments that might work. This blocks researchers from building a knowledge base on an important approach to care, and it blocks people who prefer a trauma-based approach from accessing care that may be more helpful to them than learning to manage their emotions.

When I asked Clare Shaw what she thought about the diagnosis of complex PTSD, she told me that in recognising the role trauma may have played in people's lives, this diagnosis was an improvement on the gendered and stigmatising label of BPD, but still pathologises these responses to trauma in a way that might divert attention from the enabling insight of 'just how incredibly determined and creative and hopeful people's ways of coping can be'. This is about recognising the intent behind these behaviours. Some of these behaviours may have outlasted their usefulness and some, like self-harm, may be dangerous, but by acknowledging that a person is trying to find ways to cope, you recognise their reasonableness, their resilience and, importantly, their agency. That recognition in itself can empower people to find new, more helpful ways of coping, rather than carrying internalised stigma and self-blame attached to so-called pathological personalities for the rest of their lives.

Support that empowers people diagnosed with BPD to find their way is still rare though, due to the fact that BPD is still largely believed to be untreatable.[31] But what would a cure even look like, when the behaviour, the 'personality', it describes is more reflective of the context and society a person exists within, than the person themselves? Models of treatment associated with this diagnosis are currently very limited. The main line of therapy used for BPD patients is dialectical behavioural therapy (DBT), which focuses on teaching people with a BPD diagnosis 'coping skills' in order to be able to 'regulate' their 'extreme' emotions.[32] Individuals may learn techniques for tolerating distress, recognising and regulating emotions, communicating needs, or to replace coping mechanisms like self-harm with something less harmful. In other words, coping skills for behaviours that are, in origin, coping skills.

This approach focuses on regulating behaviour that is deemed excessive, but while it may prove to be practically helpful to some, it still does not respond to what is often the original cause of the distress: abuse, violence, trauma. DBT ultimately stems from a medical view of BPD as a problem in the patient, rather than looking to potential causes in their environments that may explain their feelings and behaviour. It is, in a sense, the therapeutic equivalent of using medication to treat symptoms associated with BPD, like anxiety, depression or sleep problems, rather than addressing the underlying issue. Rather than helping people make sense of what might be confusing behaviour even to them, to understand the needs they are trying to meet, and to find new ways to respond, DBT, or drugs, only offer band-aids. In some cases, they may not even suffice as support tools, when physical safety, for example, is more pressing, or when there is such a strong sense of emotional neglect that psychotherapy is more urgent, or, perhaps, exercises to soothe the nervous system might offer more support. In the case of the women who self-harm, the response is often limited to getting them to stop doing it; the presumed irrationality of the behaviour justifies a short-sighted response that ignores the bigger picture in which those behaviours arose.

DBT is considered an evidence-based approach[33] that reliably leads to change. But the accounts of women who had gone through this form of therapy, suggest that this may have little to do with the approach itself, but rather the outcome of having any care at all. Gillian Proctor is a former clinical psychologist who, starting in 1996, worked for the NHS across a variety of services, from primary care to forensic and adult mental health. In 2013, Proctor left the NHS, as she found, increasingly, that the conditions in which she had to work compromised her values. In the last post she worked in before leaving the NHS, she facilitated a self-help group for people who self-harmed, consisting of predominantly women. In the group, women shared their experiences of psychiatric care, and Proctor noted that 'all reported having been stigmatised and just treated cruelly, especially at A&E but everywhere else as well.' Many members of the group complained about feeling restricted in what they were allowed to talk about in the context of their DBT treatment. They would be taught a so-called coping skill, for example how to regulate their anger, but, Proctor told me, 'if they started talking about an example of when they felt angry because they were thinking about the abuse they'd suffered, they were immediately shut down, told not to talk about anything personal, anything historic, and focus just on skills.' Many participants found this to be unhelpful, because it erased the context in which these emotions arose. More than that, the group found DBT to be not only delegitimising, but also overly simplistic – 'You're angry? Go hit a pillow.' Many professionals working with BPD clients echo this sense in which the approach of getting people to regulate their behaviour, to simply 'stop doing the destructive thing', misses the point, and can also be demeaning, condescending and outright harmful. At its worst, the aim of control can lead to violent treatment, involving enforced medication and physical restraint.[34] When patients are unwilling to 'comply', force is quickly perceived as a necessary measure.

'Treatment' could look very different in a system that viewed people with BPD as the survivors of trauma, and offered supportive relationships to help them understand themselves and find new options for keeping themselves safe. Unfortunately, a punitive attitude remains widespread.

This same perception carries over into the legal system, where 22 per cent of women remand prisoners in England and Wales have previously been admitted to a psychiatric hospital at some point in their lives, including 11 per cent who had been admitted to a locked ward.[35] The figure is similar in the US.[36] Compare this to less than 1 per cent of the general population who find themselves in psychiatric hospital.[37] Women who suffer mentally are being punished by a system that only sees behaviour, but does not seek to understand the reasoning behind that behaviour; and far from helping them recover, this seems to pre-empt further incarceration for many. Psychiatric labels contribute to a form of gendered policing, justifying incarceration and control. This point, of course, matters not just to women, but to anyone subjected to psychiatric treatment. We need to think carefully about what we deem to be pathological, because in a social system that allows forcible restraint on the basis of 'insanity', this is also the rationale for a form of curative violence. This violence is in actual fact antithetical to healing: people generally, not just women, are more likely to die after being detained, primarily by suicide.[38]

While BPD can be used to contain and silence anyone diagnosed with it in the psychiatric system, it can also be used as a justification for exclusion from care, because of a person's supposed 'resistance' to treatment.[39] Add to this that personality disorders in general, as an area of research and clinical treatment, have been neglected in national mental health provision, reflecting that same attitude of the early psychiatrists towards conditions deemed less severe than 'true insanity'.[40] This marginalisation of personality disorders in care was brought to light in the British context, in a 2003 National Institute for Mental Health England (NIMHE) report titled *Personality Disorder: No Longer a Diagnosis of Exclusion*. The report challenged the healthcare community to address shortcomings in the treatment of people with personality disorders.[41] In 2009, the National Institute for Health and Care Excellence (NICE) also called for specialist multidisciplinary teams and services for people with personality disorders.[42] Yet by 2011, a regional investigation found that nothing much had changed.[43] There has yet to be a systematic attempt at a national level to assess whether services have actually improved. The picture of current care provision in the UK seems bleak.

When I asked her what a more helpful response to BPD would look like, Proctor echoed Shaw's comments, emphasising that people diagnosed with BPD 'have generally found their own ways to deal with emotions, and many of the strategies people develop are much better than the skills they were taught, as in, much more effective. That's usually ignored, demeaned, seen as unhealthy and really judged.' Shaw described growing up in a family where she had to develop coping mechanisms to deal with the difficult emotions arising in her family environment. She had to find a way to process these feelings; this isn't pathological, this is survival. Recognising the human ingenuity that is reflected in behaviours that are treated as symptoms of illness in the medical paradigm, is not only more humane, empowering and helpful, it is also, simply, closer to reality.

The city of Trieste in north-east Italy has been delivering a non-medical version of care for people suffering mentally since the 1970s, which the WHO recognises as one of the most advanced community healthcare systems in the world.[44] The approach is geared towards supporting a person's suffering, rather than curing a disorder. This means that people are supported to live fulfilling lives before they reach crisis point. They are included in the city's daily activities, where citizens acknowledge the right to be different. People are at the centre; the 'illness' is put in brackets.[45] People are given access to other people, to nature, to play; in other words, they are encouraged to form their own meaningful connections with the world, which allow them to find hope, pleasure, safety, and themselves. Rather than doctors prescribing treatments to passive patients, mental health professionals work together with those who need support, to develop support that works for them.

At the core of this model is dignity and respect. Trieste has an open-door and no-restraint system of care and recovery. Of course, this isn't always easy to uphold; there are occasional situations in which people in extreme distress are temporarily detained. But the extent to which the carers impinge on a person's freedom are negotiated through conversation and compromise.[46] This takes time, and only works because it happens in the context of well-developed, trusting relationships based on collaboration, rather than controlling behaviour deemed abnormal.[47]

A similar form of contracting is seen in radical mental health groups and therapeutic communities and is slowly finding its way into mainstream care.[48] In fact, many of the tried and tested alternatives to psychiatric treatment stem from the anti-psychiatry movement of the 1960s and 70s. The anti-psychiatry movement was a reaction to the worst of the psychiatric abuse we will see throughout this book – violent forms of restraint and treatment like electro-convulsive 'therapy' and forced medication. The anti-psychiatrists pioneered new models of care, like community houses – alternatives to psychiatric hospitals that were non-hierarchical, and did not attempt to control or label people. They created places of healing, not enforced conformity.

From the beginning of the anti-psychiatry movement, survivor-led and mad-liberation movements have created a variety of alternatives to medical treatment. Often, these initiatives overlapped and were animated by other forms of resistance, all finding their answer to oppression in communal living and mutual aid.[49] There, radical alternatives moved beyond treatment or symptom management, to address the social causes of mental distress.[50] These experiments don't search for happiness or cures, as psychiatry does; they start by meeting people's bare minimum needs. The disability justice movement, for example, has developed community care and mutual aid as a response to abandonment by the state; again, simply, to survive.[51] In doing so, these were experiments in new forms of social organisation based on a social understanding of distress, and new practical ways of living and being together.

The models for care geared towards a person's well-being and functioning in the world on their own terms show what is possible when we move beyond a diagnosis of what is wrong with a person, to understand their experience. This isn't just semantics. How a person imagines their recovery, how they imagine taking responsibility for their lives, depends on how they understand themselves; on how society teaches them to understand the meaning, consequences and expectations around a borderline diagnosis.

Undeniable borderlines

It makes sense, given the history of dismissal that many women have experienced at the hands of BPD, that so many patients and researchers would prefer to see the label erased or replaced with a concept that takes seriously the causes of women's pain. It also makes sense that some have lost faith in psychiatry altogether, as a system that uses the language of pathology to demarcate those who need help from those who don't. Yet there is a tension that runs throughout this book between the need for reform – or perhaps, even, more radical overthrow of psychiatry as our dominant approach to mental distress – and the very immediate and urgent need to help people in any way possible.

Psychiatric diagnoses are the most widely known language we have for the invisible pain some of us carry, for varying lengths of time, to greater degrees. These diagnoses legitimise and communicate this pain to others. In many cases, a diagnosis will be the first acknowledgement of their suffering a person will receive, and for that reason, will often be received with relief. In some cases, even just that recognition might go a long way in alleviating their suffering. In some cases, ongoing dialectical behavioural therapy to help them adapt their behaviour to allow them to have more fulfilling relationships may be enough.

The label of BPD, however, distorts the truth. Like hysteria, the language of this personality disorder misconstrues the origin of the problem to such an extent that it often functions to control, rather than help. This is that same language that severs the connections between the problem and the world, erases the conditions that make a mind, and fixates narrowly on the emotional response of an individual that it casts as pathological – as outside the tightly policed scope of behaviour deemed reasonable. In some cases, that distortion might only amplify the sense of disconnection they feel. Where people have experienced abuse, this diagnosis that treats their behaviour rather than their abuse as the problem, may re-traumatise them, may layer on new dimensions to the self-blame and shame they already feel, and may add to the sense that they don't know themselves. It may serve to create that 'unstable self-image' that the DSM claims to drive the condition. And so, while some might turn to the blunt instrument of the label of BPD to make their distress known to the world, there are many who find that they are harmed by it.

Some argue for abolishing the diagnosis; others find it helpful. Some worry that a total rejection of the psychiatric label of BPD will harm those for whom this is a potentially life-saving and necessary route to help. Without diagnosis, they ask, how will we distinguish between people who experience distress so intensely that they use self-injury to cope and those who do not?[52] We need to ensure that the intensity of the distress and severity of a person's symptoms or emotions do not distract from the content of their experiences, which point to real abuse and violence that can only be resolved through social change.[53]

At the same time, we also need to avoid invalidating those who experience physical and mental distress currently classed as BPD.[54] This is especially important for people with intersectional identities, who will have a distinct experience of accessing support. Here, the balance of value versus harm of diagnosis might differ. A Black woman with BPD, for example, may struggle to get help because of the association of BPD with White female volatility.[55]

Where medical diagnosis is the basis for access to treatment, and, in this society, also the basis for a sense of legitimacy for those suffering from extreme pain, an outright revolution of psychiatry may be useful to some, but severely damaging to others who already suffer the far-reaching consequences of discrimination.

While this argument for prioritising access to medical care and normalising mental disease is convincing, and the need for a social restructuring around the needs of people and their differential needs indisputable, at the same time, we have to ask whether the diagnosis of BPD is the best tool we can use to bring to light and adequately respond to the particularities of a person's experience at whichever intersection of identity groups they occupy. Some may be better served by a label closer to complex PTSD that, as it hopefully acquires greater legitimacy in coming years, won't stigmatise them in the eyes of mental healthcare professionals. Some may argue that we need to push for a more multi-faceted response, beyond medical treatment alone, that may require a non-medical language. There is no straightforward answer, but a good place to start is to stop focusing solely on treating behaviours, and instead look at the root causes that we actually have evidence for; not genes or personality defects, but the abuse and trauma that is undeniably linked with borderline personality disorder.

4

The Blurred Lines of 'Female' Diagnoses: Postpartum Depression

'Baby blues' is well known as a widespread and common part of childbirth. It is a passing affliction that takes hold of many women, about 85 per cent,[1] in the immediate aftermath of pregnancy. The symptoms are emotional. They include 'crying for no reason', 'irritability', 'restlessness' and 'anxiety',[2] and they usually resolve on their own. While the exact mechanism remains mysterious, the onset occurs immediately after childbirth, and so it seems obvious that the experience of baby blues is tied to this biological event. Besides, it wouldn't be the first case of erratic emotions to be closely associated with the female reproductive system. The connection is almost implicit, so well known that it doesn't require evidence.

From this perspective, it might strike us as outlandish and nonsensical to hear that men can experience baby blues too. Postpartum depression (PPD), a more debilitating and longer-lasting medicalised cousin of baby blues, occurs in around 10 per cent fathers[3] compared to around 7–20 per cent of mothers.[4] How, we might wonder, could men possibly experience a condition that is so inherently tied to the biology of people with uteruses? Many in the medical profession would have us believe this is not just inane, but downright impossible. Impossible, that is, only from within a paradigm that presents baby blues and post-partum distress as a biological inevitability, exclusively connected to a woman's reproductive system.

If men feel depressed too, in the aftermath of the birth of their children, what other factors are driving parents into distress during and after the birth of a child beyond the biological? And could this suggest that a mother's depression isn't such an inevitability after all?

The existence of postpartum depression in men holds a mirror up to the societal and cultural assumptions framing our understanding of women with the condition. Their existence casts into question the naturalised association between childbearing and distress, and so creates an opportunity to revisit its causes, and the appropriate response. There has been a resistance in the psychiatric profession to conceding that men can have postpartum depression too; nonetheless, perhaps spurred on by media attention,[5] there is a growing research interest in paternal PPD. Many of these reports frame paternal PPD as an example of the psychiatric neglect of men. But this side-lining of men is done in relation to the positioning of women. Studying how PPD has been framed in the case of women compared to men, the types of explanations and arguments used, opens up a new way of understanding the causes of PPD – and mental distress – in general. We get a view on PPD that has less to do with natural biology, and more with the gendered, parental roles we ascribe to men and women. Why *can't* men have postpartum depression? Maybe it's far less to do with bearing children and is instead because postpartum has been defined in a social context that dictates what mothers and fathers can be and should do.

Postpartum depression, or perinatal depression, depending on if the onset of symptoms occurs during or after pregnancy, differs from baby blues in that it reflects the judgement that a woman's fleeting depression has escalated into a more chronic and debilitating condition. Her emotions now interfere with her ability to conduct daily activities, and last for longer. And yet, it reflects the same sleights of hand that simultaneously diminish and medicalise the experience as just a 'normal' part of childbirth, which afflicts most women and is easily accepted as biologically tied to being a woman.

Maternal PPD, however, is not very well understood, and is barely investigated as an experience in its own right. The DSM criteria for PPD are, in fact, the same as those for 'normal', major depression. The only difference is that the onset of symptoms must occur during the course of pregnancy or within four weeks after giving birth,[6] and last for at least two weeks.[7] The perinatal or postnatal aspect adds another dimension, a kind of qualifier, to the diagnosis, but the diagnosis itself is rooted in generic symptoms clustered around research and the experience of people with depression unrelated to childbirth. Studies on women's reported symptoms, however, show that the actual experience of PPD differs considerably from the medical definition. Women diagnosed with PPD report that their symptoms do not decrease steadily, as the DSM states they should, their sleep is not disordered but just deprived, and that their guilt is not a generalised guilt as is stated in the DSM but is specific to the fear of harming their babies due to their distress; they do not want to die, and they do not lose interest in previously pleasurable activities, but actually long for activities and feel that engaging in them would have been helpful.[8] Postpartum depression seems to describe an experience that is altogether different from those described by the DSM's broad and general category.

The postpartum experience is more than a qualifier to major depression, but seems to mean something different altogether. But this understanding is missing from the DSM. It leaves us with the same sense as the baby blues – that PPD is pathological, yet somehow is not in need of a real explanation.

We also see the same close link to a woman's biology that, contrary from opening up questions for thorough research, does away with the need for more detailed explanations, or a better understanding of women's experience. This is how it is only in the 2013 fifth edition of the DSM that postpartum depression was reclassified as a form of depression with a 'peripartum' onset. This amendment was supposed to reflect a growing consensus across research that depression for pregnant women does not always start after childbirth, but that in at least half of the cases it begins *during* pregnancy. Maternal peripartum depression can last from six months to a year, although some say it lasts for years.[9] This modification begins to cast into question, or at least complicates, that assumed link between the event of childbirth and PPD in women. There is, at the very least, a more multi-dimensional process involved.

A biological inevitability

Much of the research on PPD posits that it is caused by sudden changes in the concentrations of the ovarian hormones oestrogen and progesterone following childbirth.[10] During pregnancy, oestradiol (a type of oestrogen) and progesterone levels can rise significantly. Three days postpartum, these hormones drop to normal levels.[11] This provided a clear biological event that researchers hoped would explain the onset of PPD, and it mapped perfectly onto the understanding of the role hormones played in women's biology more generally, determining everything from their fluctuating moods to their bone density.

Scientists have worked relentlessly over the past century to prove that our gender is connected to our body. Since 1960, testosterone and oestrogen have become the most extensively used drugs in the history of medicine.[12] But the concept of 'sex hormones' gained popularity much earlier, around 1908, during the time when, in the USA and Europe, debates about the rights of homosexuals and women emerged. The idea that the public sphere was by definition masculine was so deeply engrained in the social imaginary that many scientists were arguing that women who aspired to citizenship rights had to be masculine. The next phase of hormone research was launched during the 1920s in what came to be called the 'endocrinological gold rush'.[13] Later, genetic researchers joined the effort to establish a biological basis for binary sex, through hormones. 'Sex hormones', we now know, are actually not sex-specific (men and women naturally produce and need both testosterone and oestrogen), affecting most, if not all, the body's organ systems (including the brain, lungs, bones, blood vessels and liver). All the way through, however, scientists have clung to a gender binary; even when their evidence challenged what they knew, they struggled to reconcile experimental data with what they felt certain to be true about sex differences. Even when they kept finding 'male' hormones in female bodies, for example, they never gave up the idea that hormones are essentially linked to maleness and femaleness.

Really, these so-called sex hormones should be renamed 'steroid hormones'.[14] This may have led researchers to investigate the role they play in the body more generally, but also to understand that these hormones are just one among a number of components that are important for the creation of male, female, masculinity and femininity: environment, experience, anatomy, and physiology all contribute to the patterns of behaviour we see and decide to render scientifically meaningful.

With the discovery of sex hormones, the focus may have shifted away from uterus and ovaries, but the aims of scientists remained unwavering long after hysteria was popularised. Hormones became part of ever-expansive theories that connected sex development of the gonads to behaviour and the brain. The sex hormones in the womb were assumed to lead directly to corresponding genitals and physiological traits, even including sexual orientation, cognitive patterns and interests. Gendered assumptions about behaviour were connected to biology to build an increasingly robust social division between the sexes.

In this way, hormones mapped onto and reinforced the same gendered model in medicine that made women defective and their bodies controllable through drastic interventions. Hormones were linked to female behaviour and negative traits such as weakness, mania and hysteria. For a long time, the womb and the ovaries had been considered the seat of 'undesirable' traits, like mood changes around menstruation, the symptoms of hysteria, or the evils of masturbation. In the late nineteenth and early twentieth century, removing a woman's ovaries was considered a cure to madness, and at the same time consolidated a medical justification for the control of women's reproductive systems. In the 1930s, the long-standing practice of ovary removal was replaced with a new set of hormonal therapies designed to treat an ever-expanding list of female disorders.[15] Premenstrual syndrome (PMS) was defined at this time – and, as we have seen, to this day remains associated with the idea of a biologically irrational female. Hormones became drugs that were simply looking for diseases, used to treat what were deemed abnormalities because they deviated from implicit assumptions about normal, gendered behaviour.

The long history of biologically differentiating genders underlies solely hormonal explanations of PPD. If a woman experiences 'complications', like depression, it is easy to convince ourselves that it's just a natural problem of her biological function.

But researchers have now suggested that people who experienced childhood trauma, particularly emotional abuse, are about 6 times as likely to experience PPD – unlikely to be a coincidence, that is, if we consider depression to be a normal response to traumatic experiences.[16] Professor Paola Dazzan is a professor of Neurobiology of Psychosis at King's College London and works clinically as a perinatal psychiatrist. Dazzan and her team have shown how childhood trauma in combination with stress during pregnancy significantly increases the chances of PPD for women.[17] When I spoke with Professor Dazzan, she used the case of postpartum psychosis as an example of the limitations of purely biological explanations of mental distress. While the condition, like postpartum depression, arises within two weeks of giving birth, and is tied, in this way, to a biological event,[18] it is also clear that biology does not explain the full picture. Not all women who give birth experience psychosis. Some get depressed. Some don't experience either. Depression among adoptive mothers on receiving their baby occurs at a similar rate to mothers who give birth.[19] This alone should tell us that there have to be other, environmental factors at play.

Overall, a recent review of the status of research into the biological causes – 'biomarkers' – of PPD concluded that 'there are strong inconsistencies in various findings regarding [biological] predictors and biomarkers of PPD.'[20] From the significant body of research into biological causes that has been done, the authors write, 'no biomarker is ready for clinical use today.'

The view that hormones are the driving engine of a woman's moods is so deeply entrenched, it seems common sense. But medical studies over the years have failed to corroborate the view that these hormonal changes are an all-encompassing cause of PPD, even if it is one among several other factors that can increase susceptibility. In fact, biological research has been moving steadily away from a focus on oestrogen and progesterone, and instead is considering how these hormones affect other biological processes in the body, like stress-hormone levels,[21] and interact with other social and environmental factors.

Biological factors cannot be understood in isolation, and out of context. Explanations that look to stressors in the environment offer the most hope in identifying and supporting women with maternal PPD. While decades of research have not produced one specific biological or chemical factor that causes the development of MPPD, fatigue and perceived level of stress are proven, strong predictors.[22] The reductive, gendered model of thinking about hormones perpetuates the kind of reductive thinking about women's distress across so many psychiatric disorders, which doesn't seem to give attention to the causes that lie *outside* their bodies.

When we look to the social environment, we may, once again, begin to see how women are responding to life's stressors. Rather than looking to a woman's life history, or the conditions that might be making motherhood difficult for her, the biological model situates the cause solely in the woman's body, excluding the context that helps us understand the very particular difficulties she faces that are likely to lead to depression. These explanations don't just place the cause of distress, inaccurately, in the mother's body, they also put almost all the responsibility to deal with the distress on the mother. As with hysteria or borderline personality disorder, when we look at the social pressures connected to being perceived as female in contemporary society, new common-sense explanations come into view. As the psychology professors Lisa Held and Alexandra Rutherford put it: 'When the most important job in the world becomes one of the most distressing, perhaps we need to look seriously, not only at the mother, but at the job itself.'[23]

The myth of motherhood

Biological explanations reign supreme, but the biological event of birth coincides with another milestone moment: the onset of motherhood. Motherhood sets high expectations for women. Our culture is rife with stories about how mothers should be, from the myth of maternal instinct[24] to the 'myth of maternal bonding', which sets the societal norm that mothers bond deeply and immediately with their baby.[25] These myths are useful, if we want to naturalise the societal expectation that mothers should be able to care for child, family, husband, self and work easily and without complaint.[26] They help bolster social roles. They also make failure almost inevitable. In western culture in particular, women are often placed in a dichotomy of good or bad mother,[27] creating expectations that women are judged by, and that they come to internalise and judge themselves by. A 'good mother' is limitlessly available and loving, self-sacrificing and consistently able to manage the overwhelming demands of an infant, or the family, without ever asking for help.[28] If a woman is not a good mother, then she is a bad mother. There isn't much in between. The first way to be a bad mother is to not be euphorically happy about it.[29] But there are plenty of other ways to fail. Failing to meet your child's every need, failing to return to your former physical appearance after childbirth, failing to balance work and baby without getting stressed. *It is very difficult to be a good mother, and easy to be a bad one.*

It is very plausible, from this perspective, that a mother's distress during and after childbirth could be linked to having experiences that are inconsistent with what she is led to believe motherhood should be like,[30] leading to a sense of personal failing when she believes she is unable to meet expectations.[31] This doesn't mean that postpartum depression is more common for first pregnancies; sometimes having multiple children presents new challenges, or women may receive less support, as their family assumes that they'll have less trouble with subsequent children. Indeed, just like any form of depression, having previous experiences makes you more vulnerable to recurrent symptoms. In any case, how a woman interprets her situation and capabilities is determined by the messages she has received throughout her life and in her present environment. Depression, in this sense, might very well be a result of the things that happen to mothers, and how a woman relates to them.

This feminist perspective of PPD acknowledges and validates women's experiences of motherhood. Drawing on women's own accounts, it foregrounds the changes that come with having a child, like adjusting to a new role, or difficulties breastfeeding or complications during labour when women are told this should be easy and intuitive, feelings of incompetence, the difficulty of managing contradictory advice, struggling with a lack of medical or partner support, isolation, fear about not loving a baby as much as a 'good' and intuitive mother should, and accepting a change in body image, sexuality, personal space and time, or professional and social identity, especially when it is largely felt that non-birthing partners are able to continue their lives as before.[32]

Not just the environmental stresses, but women's relationship to these demands determines if she will experience MPPD.[33] Given all the changes associated with motherhood, feeling sad, uncertain and unsettled after having a child should be normal and expected. But not according to the myth of motherhood, which implies that just to be an ordinary devoted mother, a woman not only has to sacrifice herself to her children, but also be happy about it.[34] This is often unrealistic – and undesirable. Women may well want to care for their child, may be entirely happy about having a child, and *at the same time* feel sad, distressed and grieving for their numerous, very real, losses.[35]

There is no room for this kind of complexity in the dichotomy of good and bad mother. Being unhappy, despite wanting to be happy, indicates a shortcoming that mothers are not allowed to admit to. Not just this, but research is showing that women experience a much wider range of emotional distress than the focus on depression, and sometimes psychosis, that the psychiatric literature implies. From anxiety to adjustment disorders, and through a range of psychological processes from guilt to distancing to self-blame, there is such a diversity of experience that can only be understood through research that continues to investigate how women relate to the change of motherhood.[36] But these experiences aren't really studied, and so also are not normalised. This helps explain why women experiencing PPD typically wait before seeking the help they need, if at all.[37] Where knowledge is lacking, shame fills the gap.

The cultural pressures on, and cultural neglect of, mothers is a travesty, considering that both clinical studies consistently show that peripartum social support is one of the most effective ways of preventing and supporting PPD.[38] Across a range of social contexts and cultures, social support repeatedly shows to be a key differentiating variable between those parents who experience depression after the birth of their child, and those who don't. Women who perceive their social support as lacking could be as much as twice as likely to experience PPD.[39] Social support goes a long way in alleviating the isolation and pressure new parents may feel in their new role; having those challenges recognised, supported practically and emotionally, and their new social role valued, understandably helps to ease the transition into parenthood. No diagnosis of depression is really needed here, and perhaps, in many cases, medication isn't needed either, just listening and good old-fashioned, practical support.

The reverse is also true. We only have to look at the increased rates of peripartum depression among minoritised groups, to infer the damage that a lack of social support does to new parents. Studies on peripartum depression in LGBTQ+ parents reaffirm the decisive role social factors play in the onset of pregnancy-related depression. For example, studies show that PPD is more common among lesbian mothers than among heterosexual mothers.[40] Lesbian women are a minoritised group, who are more likely to encounter the social stresses that are established risk factors for PPD, including physical or sexual abuse before pregnancy,[41] lack of practical or emotional support,[42] problems in intimate relationships,[43] and stressful life events in general.[44] They are also more likely to have experienced prenatal psychiatric problems, such as depression and anxiety,[45] which are the biggest indicators of whether a woman will experience PPD.

While research into the experience of lesbian perinatal depression is lacking,[46] it is not difficult to speculate as to the reasons for these differences in prevalence. If social support makes all the difference to mothers in a heterosexual relationship, then it is clear how the conditions of a lesbian mother's life make her more prone to depression. Lesbian mothers deal not only with a potential lack of support in the role of mother within a relationship, they also face a lack of societal support, sometimes outright hostility, and almost invariably neglect. The differences between heterosexual and lesbian women in these studies were not in biological complications, but in the way that the pressures and accompanying feelings of failure that accompany motherhood in general are compounded for lesbian mothers. And the same is true, albeit with a less seismic difference, for gay fathers. PPD among gay fathers who had a child by surrogacy is around 12 per cent compared with 8.8 per cent reported in fathers in the general population. These studies similarly confirm that fathers who report that they have adequate support, whether from partners or other services, were less likely to become depressed.[47] The research into experiences of LGBTQ+ parents once again affirms that social conditions, rather than biology, are the decisive drivers of depression for new parents.

The same, is sadly true for Black and Asian women. Black mothers experience worse perinatal support than any other group. Black women are 4 times more likely than White women to die during pregnancy, birth or post-partum in the UK, and Asian women are twice as likely.[48] In the US, 87 per cent of Black women also experience a traumatic event during the perinatal period.[49] It comes as no surprise, then, that Black mothers are 13 per cent more likely to experience PPD than any other group. In the UK, Black mothers are twice as likely as White mothers to be hospitalised with some form of perinatal depression or psychosis.[50] Part of the explanation lies in the pre-existing inequalities that already make Black women and minoritised groups more likely to experience mental distress. But besides that, the lack of care, and often traumatising care for Black mothers once pregnant only makes the situation more dire. These findings suggest that the biological process of being pregnant is not in itself the cause of depression, and so, depression isn't some inevitable consequence of bearing a child. It is not a 'natural' condition for women to put up with, but a social problem that requires adequate support.

The myth of fatherhood

Once we take into account the social environment, the solution is undeniable: social support is key to preventing, and supporting people with, peripartum depression. Isolation is a key factor in the internalised sense of failure, and the very real stress that a new mother experiences. And yet, every part of the motherhood myth works to isolate her. While women who have partners who they consider to be supportive spend less time in the hospital and recover from PPD more quickly,[51] even adequate paternal support doesn't solve the problem entirely, because mothers are so often expected to be the primary parent.[52]

This historic cultural absolution of the father from parental responsibility is reflected in the silence around paternal postpartum depression. Researchers have been much less eager to investigate the effects of pregnancy on men's moods. I spoke to one of the researchers, Brandon Eddy, a professor of couple and family therapy at the University of Nevada. He started studying PPD after his wife experienced peripartum depression and he noticed a lack of support and information among medical professionals, then gradually became aware of the dearth of information on paternal PPD (PPPD), and the impact this has on couples, in particular. He discussed a palpable resistance to the subject matter among mental health professionals and researchers, with journals reluctant to publish articles on the subject. At conferences, he often witnesses directly colleagues' immediate dismissive reactions to his team's research. 'They seem triggered by it,' he said, 'it's a strong, gut reaction.'

Dr Eddy believes that the dismissal of PPPD reflects ideologies of motherhood and fatherhood, rather than scientific findings. It shows, he said, 'how parenthood is almost completely identified with the mother.' Pregnancy, in particular, is woman's domain, associated with motherhood, not fatherhood, and a father experiencing postpartum depression undermines a social structure that depends on mothers taking responsibility for childbirth. And so, Dr Eddy is frequently met with criticism that fathers do not belong in discussions about pregnancy, even from other doctors: 'You should call it something else.' The same is evident in the research Dr Eddy has begun on reactions to fathers sharing that they suffer from PPD. Much of the time, the response is to emasculate them, using language that implies they are effeminate.

In many of the papers that do dare to name PPPD, researchers nonetheless struggle to depart from a cultural framework that identifies parenthood solely with mothers. There is a substantial body of research that has focused over the past decades on showing that if a woman experiences PPD, then a man is more likely to experience PPD (and vice versa).[53] While this research may mention in passing that this could work in both directions,[54] the predominant focus has been on how the effect works in the direction from the woman undergoing pregnancy to her partner.[55] The idea that male postpartum might have an effect on the mother has been less widely investigated, overshadowed, perhaps, by the drive to explain MPPD in terms of hormonal changes. At most, more recent studies acknowledge that while there is a clear correlation between the depression of couples, the causes and direction is unknown.[56] While you could argue that in papers that investigate predominantly male PPD, there would be less attention on how fathers affect mothers, the reverse effect has not been studied and is not represented to the same degree in the literature. There is a bias here in the kinds of questions being asked, and where our cultural assumptions about parenthood lead us to look.

Parents must affect each other; this can only work both ways. Although it is definitely possible that women *seem* less affected by their partner's depression, we have also seen how women are socialised to tolerate various levels of daily violence and abuse, and to mask their emotional reactions, or risk being dismissed as 'hysterical'. In my interview with Dr Eddy, he shared an elucidating example of a couple who came to see him together. A mother had called him telling him that her partner had been struggling since they had had their first child. Dr Eddy invited them both in and used a maternal PPD screening tool to make sense of their symptoms. The father came out as well above the depression threshold, while the mother was right at the cut-off point. The mother, however, did not mention her struggles in their sessions. Over the course of their time together, the father's symptoms declined, but the mother's stayed the same. Dr Eddy wondered if the mother was choosing to table her feelings in order to accommodate her partner's distress.

Explanations of paternal PPD expose the momentous responsibility our culture places on mothers. They help explain why paternal PPD has been neglected in medical literature – as a culture, we are nowhere near as invested in fatherhood as we are in motherhood. But PPPD also reflects and draws attention to the same woman-blaming that forms the undertone of the explanations of maternal PPD; it implies that a woman has failed her partner, her child and her biological destiny, when she is unable to meet the idealised demands of motherhood. In medical screenings, the absence of the husband's support is rarely listed as the primary cause of MPPD, even though research has repeatedly shown that lack of support is more strongly correlated with PPD than anything else.

Increased awareness of paternal PPD has the potential to shine light on the social causes of PPD for people in all gender roles. Because men are not cast in the same restrictive explanations that reduce their mental and physical states to their reproductive capacity, accounts of PPPD offer a model for more balanced and realistic explanations that may include but will not be restricted to, the role of hormones and other biological factors. PPPD subverts the certainty we place in psychiatric diagnoses, exposing the social assumptions that shape them. The explanations for PPPD can be held up against those for MPPD as a mirror, demanding that we revisit our assumptions about mothers and fathers alike and also, importantly, what support should look like.

Paternal PPD is gaining recognition in psychiatric litera-ture as well as public media. PPPD remains underdiagnosed, but researchers have established some key symptoms.[57] PPPD may manifest differently than MPPD; men might not feel able to express sadness or cry, and might instead appear stressed or burnt out, may withdraw and isolate themselves, appear indecisive, cynical, irritable, avoidant, angry, self-critical, suffer from insomnia, loss of libido, and are more likely to turn to drugs and alcohol.[58]

As awareness around paternal PPD grows, however, it is becoming clear that fathers get more reasonable expla-nations of their depression than mothers. They haven't been totally exempted from the hormonal explanations that have dominated studies on women; fathers may not have the same pregnancy hormones women do, but studies are showing various hormonal fluctuations coinciding with a female partner's pregnancy. There is, for example, a growing evidence base showing that testosterone levels drop for men around the time of pregnancy, to match the level of their pregnant partner's testosterone levels, some have suggested.[59] The interpretation of these hormonal changes, however, differ in tone from those associated with women. Hormonal changes around a partner's preg-nancy are generally discussed as favourable to encouraging 'maternal behaviour', or leading to greater relationship investment in the literature.[60] It is rare – though not unheard of – for these to be discussed in relation to depression or failure to bond with the child.[61]

Overall, the explanations for paternal postpartum depression offered over the past decades, have been based largely on social rather than biological factors. Explanations point to environmental stressors, like finances, or offer a feminist analysis pointing to the pressures of the fatherhood role (though this often comes at the cost of blaming the mother). They reveal that fathers prefer therapy to drugs (who would have thought that a depressed person would prefer to address the source of their distress, rather than only contain the biological damage?), and call for future research that responds to the preferences stated by those suffering from depression.[62] Fathers are more often granted the dignity of explanations that validate their experience, because they don't suffer under a culture and history that ties their worth to their childbearing bodies. It is important that the social explanations of PPPD become a reference point for explanations of MPPD, rather than a point of contrast that reaffirm mothers' biological failure in contrast to the external, reasonable pressures men experience.

It will benefit women to have the father's role in the family supported and recognised. But it needs to come with a parallel set of explanations and support for mothers. Awareness around PPPD could serve as an evidence base that can be leveraged to alleviate women's sole responsibility for their families. There has been a push, for example, for educating doctors to screen for PPPD. Dr Eddy told me, however, that there is still a general lack of awareness around PPPD. Many healthcare providers do not know that fathers are also at risk of depression around the time of their partner's pregnancy. Screening is essential for early detection and support and has the potential to reduce the impact and duration of a depression. Screening partners will relieve pregnant women of the burden of screening for themselves while also having to take responsibility for seeking help for their partners, though there remains much resistance to this shift, perhaps because it means involving men explicitly in a 'mother's domain'.

In the US, the National Perinatal Association (NPA) does now encourage screening fathers for depression at least twice during the first postpartum year. This is a positive step, but we have to bear in mind that even screening mothers for PPD is very inconsistent in practice.[63] This is especially true for non-White women. Research consistently shows that self-reported levels of depression for ethnically minoritised groups are significantly higher than those reflected in clinical records. This is repeatedly found to be true for the US as well as the UK, among all non-White ethnic groups,[64] and reflects racist dismissiveness around reported symptoms in a generally racist healthcare system that sees Black women many times more likely to die during childbirth than White women.[65] It also reflects a failure to make screening appropriately culturally specific. Screening is far from where it has to be for women, but when it comes to men, there is not even a working, specific and reliable screening tool; researchers often use the same criteria as they do for pregnant women to assess whether a father has PPD.[66]

As we have seen, socialised behaviours mean that an experience of depression might manifest very differently for men. Recognising PPPD will require a significant cultural shift, away from a view that holds mothers accountable for the mental and physical wellbeing of both their children and partners. But by looking at PPPD, we can start to imagine a view that recognises the pressures of parenthood *in general*, encouraging care that recognises the strain of parenthood generally. Providing screening and adequate support for fathers is part of that picture. When the responsibility of fatherhood is culturally normalised and practically supported, we are moving towards a society in which parenthood is no longer exclusively a woman's domain, and perhaps even a society in which parenthood is not an excuse for scaling back social support structures. Just as paternity leave is also an essential feminist issue, pregnancy-related psychological complications among fathers are part of shaping an equitable society, and a more developed social support system.

Not only does this view make social sense, it is a more effective approach in the context of therapeutic support for new parents. Dr Eddy told me that he typically involved both parents in therapy, even when only one of them presents with depression. This is a systems approach, where the couple defines a mutually supportive structure together. Finding that support structure is important for the person diagnosed with depression, but the process of developing a plan together is already a significant step in that direction. In fact, the ritual of turning to each other in a context where they know they'll be listened to, this deliberate choice to reflect on, and work on the relationship together, is very much part of the solution. This act of planning will reassure parents that they are supported, first by the therapist, and then, as they talk, by each other. This is an important example of how we heal by coming into relationship with each other, rather than in isolation, as an individualised problem. This means including whoever is involved – both parents, of whichever gender, or in the case that a single parent has depression, that parent and their support network, as well as any social support services – in developing the supportive structures that will hold them. We cannot treat individuals, we have to treat them in relation to the world that holds, or fails to hold, them. That includes the gender-specific cultural pressures and physical stressors they face, and it includes the people who surround them, who in turn, will require support.

This is also a good model for the 'disorders' we have seen so far, because it reminds us of the fundamental role that so many non-medical factors, like social support, play in wellbeing. The social explanations needed to make sense of PPPD, in a medicalised context that has defined MPPD, pushes the boundaries of what these biological explanations and treatments can offer. What might start as legitimising PPPD as a psychiatric diagnosis, might, in the long run, be part of an effort to show how medical tools can only go so far in meeting the challenges people might face through their lives.

5

Psychiatric Impossibilities: Psychopathy

Psychopathy* is characterised by a constellation of personality and behavioural traits that, cynically, offer many advantages to perpetrating crime. Without the ability to feel empathy or remorse, and the callous equanimity with which they hurt others as a means to an end, a psychopath is truly an extraordinarily damaging perpetrator, willing to take risks without the concern of consequences, however impulsive, and always motivated by a self-indulgent goal.

This also makes for an excellent CEO.

In his 2011 cult classic, the journalist Jon Ronson popularised the understanding that psychopathy was pretty much an essential qualification for any high-ranking business person or politician. As the New York psychoanalyst Steven Reisner puts it: 'In today's America, narcissism and sociopathy are *strategies*. And they're very successful strategies in business and politics and entertainment.'[1] We see them celebrated, with a hint of thrill and fear, in films like *American Psycho*. Here, a sleek, attractive investment banker expertly pulls off murders, his clear, detached mentality also allowing his psychopathic traits to go unnoticed

---

* While officially called antisocial personality disorder (ASPD) in the DSM-5, 'psychopath' is still widely used in the literature, and so I will use this term here.

by his wealthy colleagues and friends. He's so good that he can't seem to get arrested, even though, by the end, he realises that he actually wants to be punished.

Popular culture, then, recognises that psychopathic traits are as prevalent in our boardrooms as our prisons. In research too, a growing body of psychologists and psychiatrists are arguing that when it comes to psychopathy, CEOs and prisoners are just the most high-profile cases on a spectrum. Psychopathic traits, they say, are dimensional, triggered by all sorts of lifetime factors, and many of us have the propensity for psychopathic behaviour; it exists across the population at large. Yet virtually all psychiatric research on psychopathy has centred on male convicts. This research is justified on the premise of some glaring statistics like the 93 per cent of (male) psychopaths in prison, jail, parole or probation (more measured estimates put the rate at 20 per cent).[2] These figures can only be very approximate, given psychopathy has not been rigorously studied in the general population. There is therefore no accurate way of knowing just how many psychopaths have never been incarcerated.[3]

Justifications for this overt focus on prison populations rest on data about the propensity for violence associated with psychopathy which makes it one of the costliest of all psychiatric disorders, with estimates in the US nearing $460 billion a year; twice the cost of smoking and obesity.[4] Psychopathy, according to these reports, is also infamously untreatable.[5] Once caught, psychopaths continue to pose a high risk of prison violence, often emerging as inmate leaders.[6] Despite therapeutic efforts in prisons, once released, these people are between 4 and 8 times more likely to reoffend than non-psychopaths.[7] No wonder that psychopathy has become one of the most widely valued clinical constructs of the criminal justice system in this bleak dead-end diagnosis that seems to condemn its bearers to a lifetime of criminality.

The tests and measures used to identify psychopaths have accordingly been devised mainly to manage and mitigate the risk these people pose to society – from personality tests, to brain scans, they aim to identify and delineate a population that is resistant to treatment,[8] rather than understand and help those who are diagnosed.

This reasoning is persistent throughout the psychiatric response to other personality disorders, such as histrionic personality disorder or borderline, where the supposed danger its sufferers might wreak on society becomes a justification for violence, from forced medication to restraint, but in the case of psychopathy, persistently framed in a criminal context, the severity of control is amped up a notch. 'Criminal behaviour' is actually a diagnostic criterion for psychopathy, and so society cannot afford to waste time on ineffective cures, has to prioritise diagnosis and mitigation above all things; the choices are reduced to a simplistic binary of mass endangerment or prison for life.

And yet, for all its efforts to contain, psychiatry has missed so much. Trying to simply identify these dangerous individuals has led researchers of psychopathy down a very narrow path. Their focus solely on criminal populations has removed the study of this condition from the world in which it originates. Their directed samples have led them to develop measures that seem only, barely, to work within pre-selected populations of male prisoners. And, as is a recurring theme in the story of a profession more interested in schematising than listening, they have foregone opportunities to understand the real impact on people's lives and on the lives around them.

The female psychopath

While popular culture recognises the existence of psychopaths at the upper echelons of society, in psychiatric research, psychopathy is still understood as predominantly a male and criminal disease, and their research samples reflect this assumption. Studies continually reaffirm that psychopathic traits are more common among specifically male prisoners: 15–25 per cent of male offenders, as opposed to around 10–12 per cent of female offenders.[9] Though, again, this seems like a bit of a foreclosed conclusion, when studies have been conducted predominantly on this particular sample of the population.

The initial psychopathy scales were primarily developed and tested on a prison population of men in British Columbia by Robert D. Hare. The Canadian psychologist developed the Psychopathy Checklist (now called the PCL-R) in the 1970s, and a revised version is still often considered the gold standard for testing for psychopathic traits.[10] The PCL-R measures the scale of emotional detachment someone might have, such as their willingness to manipulate someone to a desired outcome regardless of the consequences, or their antisocial behaviour, such as aggressive or impulsive choices that might be violent or involve abruptly abandoning responsibilities. These criteria are then applied in non-institutionalised samples, including women and children, in several countries. The same test is applied to people in an entirely different context experiencing different pressures, and so likely turning to different behaviours. This is where the problem proliferates.

Dr David Cooke is one of a growing number of researchers to have challenged the standardised psychopathy measures. Given that women are less frequently incarcerated than men, here it is especially obvious that clinicians would need to be able to identify psychopathy outside the prison walls. Cooke began work on developing a more gender-sensitive scale with his colleague Elham Forouzan in the early 2000s. I spoke to Cooke to find out what had motivated him and Forouzan to develop new measures. How did they even notice that the existing measures fell short?

Cooke told me how their interest in gender differences had flowed from the cross-cultural comparisons of psychopathy he had conducted, where he had shown biases in diagnosis of psychopathy in male convicts across cultures. It started when he found a much higher prevalence of psychopaths in US samples than in Scottish samples.[11] This led him to work with colleagues to conduct a study comparing the diagnostic validity of the screening version of the PCL-R (PCL-SV) in an Iranian sample of prisoners, compared to a standardised western sample. They found that one factor, arrogant and deceitful interpersonal style, proved to have less diagnostic power in Iran; it did not differentiate between psychopaths and non-psychopaths. This is one dimension of psychopathic traits, alongside deficient affective experience (like a lack of remorse or guilt), and impulsive and irresponsible behaviour. Cooke's Iranian colleague Dr Seyed Vahid Shariat explained to him that this difference could be explained by the cultural phenomenon of *taarof*, which comprises a kind of colourful performance of respect. *Taarof* is, for example, exercised when shopping: the customer hears a standardised response when requesting a price: 'It's worth nothing,' they'll hear. This says that the seller respects the customer more than the object, not that they want to give it away for free. The customer should repeat the request for a price and thank the seller for their politeness. Another example might be that people invite anyone to their home before saying goodbye; this isn't a genuine invitation, but a display of respect. *Taarof* is a culturally acceptable manner and by no way is perceived as superficial or deceitful in Iran, but they check the boxes on superficial interpersonal style on the PCL-SV, designed based on, it turns out, a concept of psychopathy that is culturally specific.[12]

The cultural differences he found made Cooke question the validity of the concept of psychopathy in general: if diagnoses differed so much between cultures, what did psychopathy actually mean? What were the widely used and established scales measuring? If symptoms communicated something different in one cultural context as opposed to another, did they reflect the same underlying condition at all? This got Cooke and Forouzan thinking that if culture affected how people expressed symptoms, gender might, too. As with culture, they had to think about the *meaning* of the symptoms in women as opposed to men, to understand whether there was some shared pathology to speak of, and, also, to understand if this entity called psychopathy was really captured by the measurements used in the field at all.

Elham Forouzan worked at the Institut Philippe-Pinel, a psychiatric hospital in Montréal. She is Iranian by birth, raised in Paris, and perhaps this international background made her sensitive to the complexity of encompassing vastly different worldviews. She called for an overhaul of the PCL-R approach – they had to go 'back to basics',[13] she argued, and interview clinicians working with people who were thought to be psychopathic, to ask them about differences they noticed in the way symptoms were expressed.

On collecting these responses, Forouzan found that there were palpable differences between the male and female subjects diagnosed with psychopathy.[14] Looking at the affective, interpersonal and behavioural characteristics of psychopathy in females, based on twenty-five clinicians' evaluations and observations of female detainees in a provincial correctional service of Canada, she showed that, although most features reported in male psychopathy could be identified in psychopathy in females, there were key differences in how the traits were expressed, in how severe the disorder had to be to be noticeable, and in the psychological significance or meaning of certain behaviours across gender.

Her findings have since been replicated. Psychopathic women tend to show more emotional instability, verbal abuse, and manipulation as well as aggression in their family relations, while psychopathic men display more criminal behaviour and instrumental violence.[15] The research starts to show how psychopathic behaviour reflects the same gendered socialisation as behaviour in general. People with psychopathic tendencies draw on the social repertoire by which they are recognised and understood; women turn to the socially sanctioned modes of behaviour to enact their self-interest more effectively. These gendered expressions are motivated by similar rewards, namely power over others and glorification of the self, but will emerge in relation to social roles that are learned and enforced in various, complex ways.[16]

Like the cross-cultural research, the studies on gender differences show that we can't make much sense of psychopathic behaviour outside the context that gives behaviour its meaning. This has meant that the measures designed to measure psychopathy in criminal populations have proven much less effective in identifying psychopathic traits in the general population. Most items on the PCL-R, after all, aim to measure criminal behaviour. These items may not be relevant to non-criminal populations. People who have not (yet) been criminalised may exhibit core psychopathic traits such as superficial charm, manipulativeness, and lack of empathy, but not obviously antisocial or criminal behaviour. They may be less obviously impulsive. Class may also make a difference; someone who has an accent associated with education and social status might be able to mask their behaviour – high-powered business people and politicians are some of the most adept at this. This means that the PCL-R is ill-equipped to identify people with psychopathic traits in the general population. And so, we get estimates that just 1 per cent of noninstitutionalised adult men are psychopaths, compared to the obscenely high 93 per cent of adult men in prison.[17] The tests seem rigged to reaffirm this seismic schism.

Methods like the PCL-R only feed already existing popular culture claims that a psychopathic brain can be identified via imaging. These ideas contain the assumption that there is a threshold that separates psychopaths, these cold and callous archetypes, from the rest of us. This is a familiar disavowal that psychiatric diagnosis can facilitate: distancing ourselves from the abnormal, while reifying the 'norm'. Perhaps this makes for a comfortable delusion, allowing us to evade our own capacity to behave selfishly, for example. But we need to ask whether our measures and aims in identifying psychopaths are more about reifying a perceived difference between us and them, and so, an existing status quo, than they are about helping those affected.

A male, criminal disease

Psychopathy, for a long time, has been contained safely inside prison walls. There seems to be a resistance in the field of psychiatry to confront psychopathy in its proper context; to understand how the traits associated with this personality disorder might emerge in the general population. It is much easier, of course, to criminalise.

This is especially true, and especially insidious, for populations who are already criminalised. Black people are generally more likely to have psychological pain interpreted through the lens of criminality. Today, the United States has the highest rate of incarceration in the world.[18] Despite collectively making up only 29 per cent of the US population, Black and Latinx people comprised 57 per cent of the US prison population in 2016. To explain these disparities, we have to look at the way Black men, in particular, are criminalised throughout their lives. Black men are discriminated against at every stage within the criminal legal system – from being overpoliced, given harsher sentences, and disproportionately denied parole, to being sentenced to death and executed at higher rates – and prosecutors' actions and decisions are arguably the driving force behind these racial disparities.[19]

From this perspective, psychopathy lends itself to consolidating a dangerous narrative. While it is defined as a disorder, its symptoms, like superficial charm and manipulativeness, spurred on by cultural representations, are more likely to be interpreted as superpowers; to be met with fear, rather than sympathy. This has made the diagnosis, and the PCL-R, a tool used in criminal convictions. Prosecutors generally see psychopathy as a sign of an inherently threatening personality, making them more likely to push for retributive justice, while judges perceive psychopathy as associated with an increased risk of future offense, and reduced chance of rehabilitation.[20] The conflation of psychopathy with criminality provides a sleight of hand that can be used to reinforce and build on existing stereotypes of Black men as dangerous. When we consider the high percentage of supposed psychopaths in prisons (even in the UK, it is estimated that about 50 per cent of the prison population meets the criteria for ASPD),[21] we can see how maybe we are reinforcing existing stereotypes by failing to question what we are measuring: criminality, or the consequences of discrimination?

By setting the rates of Black male criminalisation along the supposed rates of psychopathy in prisons, we start to see another dimension of this convenient narrative; how psychologising is tied, for certain groups, to criminalisation. The idea that psychopathy is evil rooted in individuals lends itself to a racist narrative that certain populations are inherently criminal, rather than criminalised.

On the flip side, we can also see cultural assumptions, rather than an interest in better care, in the cases where psychopathy doesn't seem to register at all. Ever since the first efforts to measure psychopathy, discussions of gender differences and similarities were included but never properly investigated; women were only ever considered as an afterthought, perhaps relegated to a footnote.[22] It is as if, in the words of the clinical forensic psychologist Caroline Logan, who works extensively with female prisoners, 'women are treated as "funnily shaped men".'[23]

There seems to be a resistance to diagnosing women as psychopaths. The other psychiatric labels we have seen have, like HPD and BPD, very much flowed from cultural ideas of feminine normality. In these cases, gendered interpretations of behaviour seem to have trumped understanding of people's experience of distress. Psychopathy, though, remains relatively devoid of women.

When women *are* diagnosed, though, we begin to recognise the familiar impulses to pathologise non-gender conforming behaviour we have seen with the other labels. As things stand, a psychiatrist's willingness to diagnose or perceive psychopathy often seems to fall along lines of normalised gendered behaviour – when behaviour crosses these lines, it becomes much easier to cast a person in the stigmatising light of psychopathy. We only need look at a study that contrasted two case studies of women with high levels of psychopathic traits, to see how clinicians are misled by their gendered ideas about 'normal' female behaviour when diagnosing psychopathy. In the study, one female patient, Amy, presented with prototypical 'masculine' psychopathic traits (i.e., grandiose, physically aggressive, antagonistic); whereas the second patient, Bella, presented more with what might best be characterised as 'feminine' psychopathic traits (i.e., using sexuality to manipulate, aggression towards family and friends, behavioural control). The researchers only identified Amy as psychopathic.[24] Feminine forms of callousness did not register in this male-gendered diagnosis, revealing, once again, that psychiatry's diagnoses are not objective categories, but interpretations made through (unacknowledged) lenses coloured by cultural views, personal biases, and, as ever, guided by ideas of a 'norm' rooted in a gendered worldview.

Studies like these begin to reveal just how tenuous and riddled with uninspected assumptions the concept of psychopathy is. Without proper consideration for the context of behaviours, their 'meaning' cannot become clear. This context includes a culture invested in gendered ideas of normality. But this context doesn't just inform what someone's behaviour is supposed to code, and achieve, it also determines how it will be interpreted by a psychiatrist. This is equally true for a clinician's interpretation of men's behaviour. A 'symptom' like material dependency, where a woman who reports relying on her husband, falls within the gendered expectations, and might be considered to be more socially and culturally acceptable for women, and so, not pathological. In a man, particularly one who, despite changing social norms in recent years, is still often expected to act as the breadwinner, this is more likely to be interpreted as parasitic and, so, pathological.[25]

We can begin to wonder how sexism and racism might intersect to form clinicians' interpretation of the behaviour. How does it manifest for Latinx women, who are often fetishised and sexualised? Or for gay or bisexual Black men, or Black lesbians, whose level of nonconformity might shape clinicians' perception of their behaviour as antisocial or aggressive in particular ways? There is sparse research on psychopathy in these groups. Some studies have suggested that ASPD, the bracket under which psychopathy has been subsumed in the DSM-5, is more often diagnosed in lesbian women and bisexual men or women, but the findings are inconclusive.[26] Again, research has focused on understanding psychopathy as an individual entity, rather than a construct that has emerged from a particular set of concerns, and in a particular cultural context. Psychiatrists have not spent much time reflecting on their own role in perpetuating social systems, and so haven't questioned whether these constructs are doing more harm than good.

The meaning of psychopathy

The research on gender and cultural differences in the presentation of psychopathic traits illuminates not only a blind spot in the field of psychopathy research but, rather more existentially, has cast its fundamental concept into question. For all the effort they have spent on trying to distil and identify psychopathy in dangerous criminals, the truth is that there still isn't a consensus on what psychopathy is.

When I spoke to Cooke about it, he admitted: 'I think we're all still struggling to try and get at the essence of this. We know there's something there because when you meet someone with this disorder, they do feel quite different from people without the disorder. There is something unusual, but we're all struggling to find a methodology for describing it.'

A big part of the problem is, he added, that researchers often conflate the measure with the disease: 'They think psychopathy is a score on a test.' The failure to diagnose women using existing measures, however, reveals the test as just one blunt instrument for getting at a concept that in itself remains very much disputed. The issue of gender and cultural bias reveals the faults in the concepts of psychiatry in general. Researchers have developed various measures for a psychopathic personality, but are trying to get a grasp of the same phenomenon, Cooke said. In doing so, they have developed different procedures, scales, and even different names – 'antisocial personality disorder is an attempt to get at a thing that we would call psychopathy. Others would call it sociopathy; others would call it social personality disorder.' Sociopathy is a term that some find less stigmatising than psychopathy, as it tends to imply that the behaviours associated with the disorder are learned, or responses to trauma, rather than a brain-based condition present from birth; different terms are used among researchers, depending on what types of explanations they are interested in. ASPD has replaced psychopathy in the fifth edition of the DSM, and places more emphasis on behavioural aspects of psychopathy, such as aggression, impulsivity, and violations of others' rights, and less on personality characteristics like callousness, remorselessness and narcissism. This is supposedly to reduce stigma, but psychopathy continues to exist as a subtype within the broader category of ASPD. Measures like PCL-R are designed to 'measure' psychopathy, generally regarded as a more severe and violent form of ASPD, although, again, there isn't really a consensus on this.[27] The problem, Cooke says, is one of measuring something undefined, and as ever, that is dangerous terrain, open to abuse in the form of knowledge claims based on flimsy ground – as the profession tries to assert its relevance despite these gaping holes. Again, this becomes even scarier knowing that assessments of psychopathy bear significant weight in determining life sentences, death sentences and other forms of punishment that target already discriminated groups of the population; all this based on a dubious, ever-shifting concept. That's why 'going back to basics', as Cooke and Forouzan proposed, is not just good science, but a matter of social justice.

Cooke himself went on to work on the Comprehensive Assessment of Psychopathic Personality (CAPP), a measure to rectify some of the issues associated with the PCL-R. While still not perfect, with the CAPP, Cooke has tried, at the very least, to pose gender differences as an open question to be investigated; to return to 'the basics', and ask what psychopathy actually is. This was necessary in the context of his research on gender differences, because without a baseline consensus understanding of psychopathy, even the best intended research comparing men and women is futile, only further entrenching misunderstanding.

The CAPP differs significantly from the original psychopath test. It does not include, first of all, criminal or antisocial behaviour as diagnostic criteria, diverting researchers' views from the tautological thinking that pretty much sees criminality as a foregone conclusion for psychopaths.[28] The CAPP includes a much broader range of symptoms and categories that help describe a person, looking at the way, for example, they relate to attachment, dominance, or their sense of self. Then, unlike the PCL-R, which is based on just one person's view of psychopathy, the CAPP uses multiple sources and methods to assess how far a subject meets its criteria. Assessments are done via interviews and are combined with 'collateral information' – information about the subject in question from their network that may also include medical records, police reports, pharmacy records, mental health, or school records – to deduce the presence of the traits that they have connected to psychopathy, but also to assess the strength of the traits. The measure is supposed to be used to help clinicians explore and compare various possibilities, taking on board all this information about the person and their social world, to consider the relative merit of these explanations. In this way, the researchers have tried to attune themselves to both the differences in gendered expressions of psychopathic traits, as well as their own gendered interpretations.

Another important difference from the PCL-R, is that this method is also supposed to allow scope for measuring changes in symptom severity; rather than the dead-end diagnosis of the PCL-R, which is designed to measure the presence of symptoms in the past one to two years, the CAPP is based on the premise, supported by research, that psychopathy is dynamic, not static or inherent, and that a person might slide up or down the spectrum according to their social conditions or treatment.[29] The CAPP test tries to build a picture of how psychopathic behaviour manifests in a person's life, and in doing so, begins to move towards describing the experiences and conditions that give rise to psychopathy.

This is a good first step for our understanding of psychopathy in general as well as in women in particular. It creates an opportunity to ask how gender roles give rise to and shape this behaviour – gender roles being an important part of the way in which any behaviour develops in our social world. But these descriptions will also counteract the illusion often given by quantified, diagnostic measures, that the experiences they supposedly capture are already understood, definitive and generalisable.

Descriptions like these, then, blur the bounds of categories, and encourage a movement away from categorisation, towards description. This is closer to an attempt to understand how an individual's experience takes shape, and so, also, a much more informed place from which to understand what they might need. But this would require an approach that is less about categorisation and containment, and more about describing, relating and expanding.

These insights are helpful in terms of including women in an understanding of psychiatry, but they are just the tip of the iceberg in terms of what attention to gender and culture can show us about 'psychopathy'. The criteria on tests like the PCL-R reflect the origins of the research on psychopathy. It was designed to predict outcomes relevant to criminal populations, like violence and the likelihood of reoffending. These outcomes aren't as relevant, or helpful, for non-criminals. But exposing the biases of psychopathy research also reveals the carceral logic driving a profession and legal system, sidestepping a real understanding of what they are even measuring at all and precluding the possibility to help. The goals for non-criminal people with psychopathic traits might not only be to predict the likelihood of a violent act. It might be more important to identify and help them with non-criminal forms of psychopathic behaviour related to their ability to work and relate to others. The PCL-R doesn't do as well with these outcomes; another test might be more fit for purpose, but the CAPP also confronts us with the limits of what a measure can do. Measures can help psychiatrists identify patterns in behaviour that help them refine their tools, but these measures are designed to shore up definitions and do fairly little to expand an understanding of psychopathic behaviour as it arises in a life lived, and so do fairly little to build a fuller understanding of the meaning of this behaviour before it is schematised or criminalised.

We need to revisit our goals of identifying psychopaths because they limit what psychiatry is able to offer people diagnosed, their communities and society at large. If the aim of clinicians is still primarily to identify criminal traits, how can we imagine care beyond incarceration and detainment? What are the societal benefits of preventative treatment? What does support for non-criminal psychopaths and their communities look like? To move beyond the prison walls may also mean investing resources in projects beyond psychiatry that respond to the impact of psychopathic behaviour in the world.

Freeing psychopathy

There is a growing consensus among mental healthcare researchers today that about 1.2 per cent of people in the general population meet the criteria for psychopathy (0.3–0.7 per cent for women and 1–2 per cent for men),[30] but as many as 30 per cent of people in the general population display some degree of psychopathic traits,[31] which may have consequences much less criminal, but nonetheless detrimental to the person and their community – relationships will suffer, and they may put themselves in risky situations, exposing themselves and others to danger. This understanding of psychopathy as a much wider phenomenon has, for one, important implications for our understanding of psychopathy in women. If it is true, as the body of research on psychopathy in women is suggesting, that psychopathic women 'use more subtle and relational ways of exploiting and dominating other people',[32] a form of aggression which takes place primarily in domestic contexts, then there is a huge proportion of violence and disturbance that is going unidentified and unsupported.

It is tempting to think that, unlike the other personality disorders that criminal systems and psychiatric institutions have eagerly leveraged against women to pathologise and contain them, perhaps in the case of psychopathy, women have escaped the bounds of this particular form of medical control. Only, when we see women's exclusion from psychopathy in the context of psychiatry as a whole, we will draw different conclusions. Perhaps women's exclusion from psychopathy simply tells us something about the gendered locus of psychiatric control. Some researchers have claimed that women with psychopathy are often misdiagnosed with borderline personality disorder. Some have gone so far as to suggest that borderline is simply a female-specific version of psychopathy, characterised by emotional dysregulation and manipulative callousness.[33] Given the logics that we have seen to drive diagnosis of women with borderline, I wonder if perhaps this is simply easier to concede. Borderline expresses that dual sense in which women are regarded as volatile and at the same time infantile and non-threatening. Perhaps this image, and its associated response of restraint in psychiatric settings, is a more 'intuitive' response to behaviour perceived as dangerous in women. Not dangerous enough for prison, but dangerous enough to be dismissed.

Black women aren't any more likely to be diagnosed as psychopathic. There is some sparse research on the disparities in diagnosis of personality disorders across ethnic minorities and racialised groups. Some research suggests that Black women are less likely to get a diagnosis for a personality disorder (PD) in White-dominant countries.[34] One analysis compared Black with White groups in US and UK, and included community, inpatient and prison settings, secure and non-secure inpatient settings, and different approaches to diagnosis. They generally found a lower rates of PD in Black women.[35] Another UK study found a lower prevalence of PD in all ethnicities compared with the White British population, and little overall variation in personality disorder diagnosis rates between Black and other minority ethnic (BME) groups.[36] The international study was particularly interesting because it suggested that personality disorders might simply be ignored in more secure settings and in inpatient settings, where so-called acute care, which might involve medication, surveillance or restraint to manage high risks, takes priority. This would reflect a situation where more Black people find themselves considered high-risk more often, justifying more 'care' comprised of risk-mitigation and enforced regimens, rather than long-term psychological support.

This again warns us against the assumption that exclusion from a diagnosis of ASPD, or psychopathy, means that women are somehow off the hook; they may simply be invisible. They may be subjected to other forms of control, or neglect. Some researchers have also explained the lower prevalence of ASPD among Black women by pointing to the racialised groups being generally less likely to access mental health services, due to either general wariness of abuse based on lived or inherited trauma, or cultural norms that discourage getting help. Others suggest that a so-called 'reverse racism' may mean that psychiatrists may be reluctant to make a diagnosis of personality disorder because it may be perceived as racist. This again indicates the work psychiatrists have to do to better understand how to work cross-culturally, as well as the work the profession will need to do to diversify its workforce. Neglect might be preferable to the control or abuse many Black people risk in encounters with the mental healthcare system, but neglect can still be fatal and is still very much a form of culturally sanctioned abuse.

Neglect masks a host of lacks: inadequate research, substandard treatment and a lack of a social care system that can support women and their communities struggling with the symptoms associated with psychopathy. These cracks become readily visible when we look at the narrow focus on prison populations that has shaped the field of psychopathy research and practice; on the other side of this fence is another form of social neglect.

The cracks, though, are also where we can make the biggest difference. The most important advances in psychopathy treatment are unlikely to happen from within the male criminal context long associated with psychopathy. Research on preventative treatment for children and adolescents outside the prison system is a real source of hope and contradicts the view that psychopathy is untreatable.[37] The most successful approaches to treating psychopathy start in early childhood. These therapies are used with children who display what are called unemotional (CU) traits, such as lack of empathy, sense of guilt and shallow emotion, that are considered to be a precursor to psychopathic traits in adulthood. When these children receive a mix of behavioural and exploratory therapy consistently and from an early age, they learn to socially adapt. Family-focused therapy is particularly effective in helping children and their families to cope. Parents work directly with a clinician who trains them to understand and respond to their child's symptoms and behaviour at home. This is more effective than either individual therapy or medication. While of course this kind of therapy isn't available to everyone, and not all families are in a position to participate in these programmes, what this shows is how important a person's community is to supporting through change; psychopathy isn't actually an individual problem, it affects all those around them in ways that incarceration doesn't address; not just that, but the whole community needs to be involved in creating a supportive environment for change. When people hold less stigmatised views of the traits associated with psychopathy, are able to talk about them, and receive adequate support to be able to support their children as well as their own needs, we find that psychopathic tendencies do not make someone inherently criminal.

Even treatment that starts later, in adolescence, helps. Even those who have already entered the criminal system, after participating in a treatment programme they are less likely to reoffend. In one study, those who didn't participate in the programme were twice as likely to reoffend as those who did. These treatment programmes are most effective when they involve structured interaction with people who model sociable behaviour and attitudes.[38] All the most effective treatment options share a combination of structured, therapeutic support, practical skills, and an organised and supported community structure.

The idea that the social environment needs to be supportive for a person to change is, then, generally reflected in the most innovative care schemes in prisons.

Chromis, for example, is a progressive treatment programme in the UK designed to reduce the risk of violence in those with high levels of psychopathic traits. Launched in 2005, it was delivered as part of the regime on a unit specifically tailored for men with high levels of psychopathic traits and other personality disorders, called the Westgate unit.[39] The model was geared towards engaging the prisoners in treatment, helping them find new and fulfilling ways to live more 'pro-socially' and achieve their goals without the use of violence. Like the family approaches at home, this model treated the whole unit, rather than individuals. It was recognised that if individuals were treated, then sent back to their wings, they'd likely relapse in these unsupportive conditions. The whole wing had to be a therapeutic environment, with staff trained to respond in a consistent way to support prisoners.

The programme was also adapted, as many cognitive and behavioural therapies for people with psychopathy are, to offer novelty and stimulation for this group of people who get bored easily. It was tailored to people's individual needs and aims and emphasised choice rather than control by working with people and maintaining a dialogue about the treatment that makes sense for them. The scheme has proven to effectively reduce self-reported anger and physical aggression.[40]

And much of this had to do with better relationships with the staff working at the prison. Having worked with uniform staff in treatment, the prisoners said they were more prepared to engage with uniform staff after completing the programme, a finding also supported by subsequent records of their behaviour. Most referred to a particular relationship that had helped them to shift their overall perception of the staff. And this makes sense; someone trying to work with them and help them, rather than control and punish, made them feel more supported and respected. This response doesn't sound pathological at all, but very human.

The success of the programme of effective support for people at the most 'extreme' end of societal risk raises an interesting possibility for psychiatric treatment more generally. Again, as with BPD, the idea that people with mental health difficulties are inherently dangerous, in this case, even criminal, easily overshadows all possibilities for care that are preventive, community-based, and not premised on control. While, of course, it is important to keep people safe from crime, conflating psychopathic traits with criminality is a dangerous, under-supported leap that becomes the basis for a punitive response that misses real needs, and opportunities to help. Again, as with BPD, it would make more sense for us to make the opposite assumption: that crime is preventable, containment avoidable, and that we ought to design our care systems with the aim of helping people find their way.

To get a better understanding of the problem, and

solutions, to psychopathy beyond the prison context, I spoke with the writer M. E. Thomas, perhaps one of the most well-known women with psychopathy, who wrote *Confessions of a Sociopath*, which was published in 2013, based on her blog, Sociopath World. In her blog, she details what life living with psychopathy is like. Thomas told me that the responses to her blog often betray a gendered dismissal: 'People don't want to accept it,' she said, comparing her experience to the reception of a male figure like the neuroscientist James H. Fallon, who wrote a book published in the same year about his discovery, through his scientific research, that his own brain scan perfectly matched the patterns he'd spotted in the brains of psychopathic serial killers.[41] 'No one seems to question Fallon,' Thomas said, and while his scientific status may play a role in granting him authority to proclaim a diagnosis, we have to attune ourselves to the ways in which his gender makes him both more authoritative, and also a more believable psychopath.

In a society where the dominant, and often the only, response to mental distress is psychiatric, not recognising female psychopathy also means that there is no support, of any kind, for the people it harms. Not for the criminal forms of violence done by women with psychopathic traits in the domestic sphere,[42] nor the 'non-criminal' harm that a 'feminised' violence does in communities, such as the trauma of family members being consistently manipulated, or the social isolation parents might experience as a result of their child's behaviour, or the very real fear of what a person, not criminal but always threatening criminal offence, might do to the people it involves. Nor is there support for the women with psychopathy themselves – who, contrary to popular belief, *do* suffer with feelings like anxiety, which may even be one of the drivers of this kind of behaviour.[43] With help, they can learn to satisfy these personal needs, forging more fulfilling relationships that will benefit everyone involved. Without help, the violence will proliferate in communities, doing most harm, as ever, where there is most need. In this scheme, women aren't off the hook, but neither are most men, of course, when swathes of males diagnosed with psychopathy are being incarcerated in a system that does little to support them.

The statistics showing the prevalence of psychopathy outside of criminal contexts, in the population at large, and in the domestic sphere, points to a problem that has not been addressed by a discipline fixated on classifications, rather than understanding. New measures to identify psychopaths are not going to cut it; we need to draw on the insights revealed by gendered patterns of prevalence, to intervene where the problem actually lies; that is, in relationships, between people, in the world.

What does it mean to 'understand' psychopathy? As we turn our minds from quantifying and controlling individuals to supporting communities, we begin to get a view of what this behaviour means in the social world we all live in. And in doing so, we build a knowledge base that is operational, that might safeguard a society from the sliding scale of human malice, much more thoroughly and sustainably than the crude tools of measurement and containment.

Bringing psychopathy home

Lisa Michael is the president and cofounder of PsychopathyIs, an organisation formed to fill the gaping hole that faces anyone dealing with psychopathy in the real world.

In order to tackle the suffering caused by psychopathy *throughout* the lifespan, they try to address the needs of those with psychopathy as well as their families and communities, through education and advocacy. They advocate for research into the causes of psychopathy and improved interventions, and they also work to improve public understanding of the signs and symptoms as it manifests in the real world.

Lisa herself is the mother of a daughter with psychopathy. When we spoke, she told me that she spent her daughter's childhood being afraid of her; that her daughter was 'ice-cold since she could talk'. Lisa didn't know what to make of her daughter's behaviour. 'I just didn't know psychopathy was a thing ... Why would I know it was a thing? I just thought ... She doesn't want to be hugged. She's not friendly to me. I don't know: I just [felt] unlucky.'

It took Lisa a long time to find recognition for her child's abnormal behaviour, which she knew exceeded the usual levels of childhood disobedience, but was dismissed by everyone around her. For a long time, this made Lisa hesitant to seek support. She wondered if perhaps she, rather than her child, was the problem. She eventually went to see various psychiatrists, to pose the question to them, but only received diagnoses for her daughter that just didn't seem to fit, until, after twenty-seven years, she found a description that seemed to make sense.

Lisa expressed her ongoing bafflement to me that in her community in the heart of Silicon Valley, that beacon of cutting-edge knowledge and innovation, no one wanted to solve this problem, let alone recognise her child's issue. Of course, given what we know about the socioeconomic gradient along which psychopaths are either celebrated or pathologised, perhaps it comes as no surprise that psychopathic traits, in this competitive economic context, could have been regarded an asset, maybe recognised instead as the early rudiments of a healthy 'go-getter' attitude that would serve her well later in life.

Lisa herself cites several possible reasons for the general failure to recognise her child's behaviour as psychopathic. Her daughter was physically attractive, 'a very pretty girl', she says, which made people predisposed to dismiss the severity of her manipulative behaviour.

A lack of understanding about how psychopathy manifests for women also seems to have played a role in the failure to identify these mental health problems in her daughter. Echoing the research we've seen, Lisa described her daughter's behaviour as emotionally manipulative rather than physically violent; she didn't create issues at school in the playground like, as she puts it, 'you might expect from a boy with conduct disorder'. It was insidious, and often went undetected. Add to all this a general misconception of what mental distress looks like. Lisa cites the idea, for example, that 'if your kid isn't doing drugs and is getting good grades, they must be fine,' echoing that by now familiar idea that mental health is measured by our ability to thrive in an unwell society.

This is all compounded, Lisa says, by a general reluctance to understand children through the lens of psychopathy. 'You can't really call a three-year-old abusive, you can just call them difficult. By the time she was a teenager, she was actually emotionally abusive, but it wasn't recognised like that.' The reference to abuse is helpful in understanding the impact 'non-criminal' psychopathy has in the world. Abuse of all kinds, usually directed at women, usually taking place in domestic contexts, is trivialised as less serious than 'real', violent crime. Abuse falls into the domestic, feminised, neglected, so it's not surprising that research on psychopathy has not prioritised this kind of harm.

Dismissal breeds silence which breeds stigma which breeds shame. Especially for the parents of children with psychopathy, this reluctance to take the condition seriously in children fosters a culture of parent-blaming. While she doesn't deny that victimisation plays a role in the psychopathic behaviour of many children,[44] Lisa also cautions against the view that it can only be the result of poor parenting, or of a parent being unable to handle normal childish misbehaviour. At its worst, the implicit feedback this sends is, in Lisa's words: 'If your kid's treating you badly, you must deserve it.' This reinforces stigma, in turn silencing parents who are afraid to raise the issue, when no one seems willing to recognise the extent of the harm this abuse causes in families and communities.

Mothers are generally seen as the primary caregivers of their children and therefore blame is disproportionately, and all too easily, attributed to them when things go wrong. A single mother is more likely to be demonised before there is any discussion of an absent father. The directing of blame towards mothers, in particular, then, is another consequence of a lack of a societal response to psychopathy. Just as a lack of understanding and support leads to criminalisation rather than rehabilitation, when no responsibility is taken on a societal, systemic level for psychopathy, parents get the blame and the burden. Lisa referenced the history of the Neo-Freudian 'mother-blamers' in 1950s America to emphasise how this can and needs to change.

In the 50s, a series of personality profiles were devised directly linking a mother's disposition or parenting approach to the problems of society, evidenced in individual children. Overprotective mothers stunted their children's maturation and were, according to a leading American psychiatrist, 'our gravest menace' in the fight against communism; excessively permissive mothers produced children who would become juvenile delinquents; a mother who smothered a son with affection risked making him homosexual; while the undemonstrative 'refrigerator mother' was blamed for what is now diagnosed as autism.[45] The profile of the 'schizophrenogenic mother' also emerged at this time and persisted through the 1970s, to refer to the mothers who had made their children schizophrenic.

This history of blaming parents, especially mothers, for their children's problems, adds another factor that helps explain the disbelief Lisa faced when talking to people about her daughter as psychopathic. In response to similar experiences, the parents of autistic and schizophrenic children formed organisations like the National Alliance for the Mentally Ill (NAMI), which still exists today to raise awareness and provide support and education where this was lacking and did much in shifting responsibility from parents to systems to support them and their children. The same needs to happen with psychopathy, Lisa says.

When Lisa finally received the information she needed to understand her child's behaviour, it helped her make sense of it, but it didn't help her deal with the pain and shock that had resulted from what she likens to an abusive relationship. There were no support systems for this kind of situation, as the reluctance to face psychopathy in the population is mirrored in the services available. Lisa contacted the psychologist and neuroscientist Abigail Marsh at Georgetown University, and they started PyschopathyIs to fill that gap.

PsychopathyIs builds on the approach of mental health organisations in the US that have promoted education and advocacy for those affected by neurodevelopmental disorders, such as Autism Speaks and NAMI. Psychopathy is not included in the remit of these bigger organisations – again, reflecting this distancing, this taboo and lack of information around behaviour that we prefer to relegate to the world of prisons. Equivalent support structures therefore don't exist for psychopathy. But they desperately need to, Lisa says, to support all those affected.

It is difficult providing care where understanding doesn't exist; it is difficult to even identify where help is needed. But this understanding won't come unless the field turns its attention to the signs and patterns that point to a particular constellation of distress in the world. And we need to keep asking ourselves what we are trying to understand, and to what end. Psychiatry has tried to distil categories, to arrive at definitive metrics to capture people perceived as psychopaths in a model for medical treatment, but is more likely to put them on a path to incarceration. We need to generate more options. We do that by prioritising care over cure, working with people and their communities to identify what is helpful to them, as we support their ongoing relationships.

Nonetheless, there exists a tension between the need for a language for people with psychopathy and their communities, and the misunderstanding this language spreads. It can be helpful to have a language that legitimises the problem that individuals diagnosed with psychopathy and their communities face. Medical language holds authority in our culture. Having a diagnosis helped validate Lisa's experience, absolve her of self-blame, and understand the nature of the problem she was dealing with. Having a terminology can help foster understanding and protect social bonds. At the same time, defining a (little understood) experience to the level of a disorder is inherently fragmenting; it separates the abnormal from the normal, and also misrepresents the actual nature of psychopathic behaviour, which, as all behaviour and experience, exists on a spectrum.

In fact, some psychiatrists have now taken on the language of formulation rather than diagnosis to describe their process. As opposed to diagnosis, formulation is instead a process of making sense of a person's difficulties in terms of aspects of their current situation, like their relationships or experiences of work, living situation, and own way of making sense of their situation, and explaining their distress. In its ideal form, this process would lead to a mutually agreed plan, not an imposed diagnosis, to deal with the difficulties. This may include resolving financial problems or learning to deal with difficulties in a relationship, and would help identify other, non-medical services to help support them in their lives. It might involve limited use of medication to target some symptoms, like lack of sleep or anxiety, but would also involve a realistic discussion of potential side effects.[46] Lots of psychiatrists already piece together a complex story of the origins and causes of a patient's problem, but what the perspective of formulation shows, is that a diagnosis might not be necessary to providing mental healthcare; we may not need a medical language, and will need more than just a medical language to come to an understanding of what is going on for a person. Alternatively, we could imagine using a few, broad diagnostic categories to describe mental *experience*, rather than mental disease. We may say, 'you're experiencing a lot of anxiety, or psychosis or depression,' rather than 'you have depression,' which might reinforce the idea that you are individually responsible, or 'you are depressed', the idea that you are pathological. If we can uphold the understanding of these concepts as broad brackets of experience, then there is room to explore what has put us in these states, and what might help us move to a more comfortable place. We can communicate about mental distress in a way that isn't pathologising or stigmatising, that is more descriptive and closer to a person's individual experience, and that may even be more informative when designing a person's care.

Once we have established a narrative of what has happened, we won't need a medical language to communicate with non-medical professionals, like social workers, community support, family and friends, to develop an appropriate plan that meets a person's aims, needs and current capabilities.[47] Again, as ever, any changes we make to our official ways of talking about mental health will need to take into consideration the clarity diagnosis brings some, and the need to support individuals in finding ways to talk about their experience and access the support they need.

A more multi-faceted language for describing mental distress and experience might also lead to different kinds of research, focused on what is helpful to people, rather than shoring up the legitimacy of a psychiatric theory. Even if brain scans and diagnostic tests do what scientists promise, it remains unclear how they will alleviate the cost to society, which extends far beyond craniums or prison walls, and deep into the family home and the community. If the cost to society is really the driving concern when it comes to psychopathy, why isn't research addressing the problems hidden in plain sight? Why aren't more scientists studying where it happens early on, finding ways to support and intervene? Responding to the violence of psychopathy in the world will require longitudinal data: studying the developmental patterns of antisocial, callous and manipulative behaviour in the population, and not just criminal populations.[48] Without these studies on the development of psychopathy in society at large, we will lack the map we need to identify where help is needed.

With research geared towards early and ongoing support for psychopaths and their communities, the help available might look very different. So-called treatments are currently limited, partly because governments have overall spent fewer resources on trying to work with, rather than shore up definitions of psychopathy; indeed, the Chromis study we saw has been discontinued due to the high cost (the potential *societal* cost of it being discontinued, unsurprisingly, goes unmentioned). And, as is a recurring issue in psychiatry, searches for career-making explanations detract from the work that can be done to help. But there are some examples of successful therapies that help people diagnosed with psychopathy manage their own behaviour.[49] There is also a growing body of psychopathic women in the population who have accepted treatment and provide useful case studies in what works: M. E. Thomas, for example, uses meditation, psychological therapy and peer-to-peer support from their online community to help manage their disorder.[50] But enacting these approaches will require narrowing the moral gap we have insisted on between society and a pathologised few, and bringing psychopathy home.

Psychopathy draws attention to the multiple lines we draw with any diagnosis. Between sane and insane, human and inhuman, us and them. We need to work hard to inter-rogate the exclusionary logics that separate us from what we are not. We need to be aware of, and take responsibility for, the discrimination we enact, so that we can make choices, as a society, in the confidence that the care we offer serves the people affected, not our own, fortified notions of who we are. The impact of psychopathy on communities, unlike the science, is undeniable. We do not need to 'explain' psychopathy scientifically to provide social support to parents, or to validate their claims – these are high-impact measures that can be taken now. Taking psychopathy seriously means accepting whatever it is as part of our social world.

6

The Biological Dream

Schizophrenia, perhaps more than any other psychiatric disorder, has come to serve as the epitome of madness. Insensitive to the stigmatising consequences for those who suffer from its symptoms, in common parlance and popular culture alike the diagnosis carries with it an image of mental chaos, a personality dysregulated and in total disarray. Throughout history, it has been relegated to the purview of villains, demons and malicious spirits. Even today, it is often perceived as a state of utter, constant and irreversible psychosis, an unravelling of all meaning. It is a place on the fringes of society, where we are not who we are and where the world is not what it is, a place that deeply threatens the core of how we understand ourselves as individuals.

This understanding, of course, is inaccurate, laden more with prejudice than truth, but there is a hint of truth to it, in that psychiatric definitions have made schizophrenia a condition that is confusing and senseless, and one that only afflicts people who have already been socially marginalised.

Schizophrenia, in the fifth edition of the DSM, is diagnosed by an individual presenting with at least two of the following symptoms: delusions, hallucinations, disorganised or incoherent speech, grossly disorganised speech or catatonic behaviour and 'negative symptoms'. 'Negative symptoms' include diminished emotional expression and avolition, the inability to initiate and persist in self-directed purposeful activities. The overall disorder, which must include at least one of these negative symptoms, needs to persist for at least six months, but may go through periods of 'residual' symptoms when the disease is only noticeable by the negative symptoms.

Taken in sum, it is possible to imagine schizophrenia in many different configurations. The loose stipulations on an impressive range of symptoms make the diagnosis incredibly flexible, and the residual symptoms particularly open up the category, drawing in people whose symptoms don't persist in the way the guide specifies they must for six months under its umbrella. This, sort of, escape clause holds together the symptoms included in the extremely broad category of 'schizophrenia'. While this might reflect the range of ways in which meaning disassembles for people, it is cause to wonder whether there is a meaningful, singular 'disease' to speak of. The psychologist John Read has shown that there are as many as fifteen ways that two people can meet the DSM criteria for schizophrenia without sharing a single common symptom.[1] The psychiatric definition, far from offering clarity on a particular biological condition, begins to echo the popular understanding of the term – as a far horizon of disassembled meaning.

Over the course of the history of schizophrenia in psychiatry, its meaning has always been difficult to grasp. Definitions of the disorder have expanded and contracted in the DSM over the years, rectifying inaccuracies with subtypes, proliferating into a kaleidoscopic blur, merging into a spectrum and differentiating out again. When viewed across decades, schizophrenia has variously been referenced as a symptom, a disorder, a group of disorders, a spectrum of disorders, and a syndrome.[2] [3] Schizophrenia has existed simultaneously as a disease and a psychogenic disorder,[4] and has appeared as a subcategory of autism and of epilepsy. It has been divided into subtypes that made appearances, then quietly faded into the abyss, included paranoid schizophrenia, disorganised schizophrenia, catatonic schizophrenia, undifferentiated schizophrenia, residual schizophrenia and juvenile schizophrenia. There has been late schizophrenia, latent schizophrenia, postpartum schizophrenic psychoses, pseudoneurotic schizophrenia, process schizophrenia, postinfluenzal schizophrenia, schizomania, schizophrenia deliriosa, childhood schizophrenia, simple schizophrenia, true schizophrenia, transient schizophrenia, systematic schizophrenias, and the modern, broad schizophrenia.[5]

The story reads like a litany of discarded diagnoses – and yet, this inability to land on a stable definition doesn't seem to have, at any point, caused us to question the underlying concept driving it all. Psychiatrists themselves remained overall unperturbed by the often quite drastic changes to their definitions of the illness, and what it actually refers to. For example, the DSM-III (published in 1980) specified that the onset of schizophrenia must occur before the age of forty-five. This rendered someone unable to be diagnosed after their forty-fifth birthday. But in the revised 'Text Revision' DSM-III-R (1987) this requirement was dropped without much discussion.[6] In fact, these changes seem to have, if anything, created a hunger for further research down this potted road, underscored by the belief that this was a process not just of redefining and revising, but refining; honing our understanding of schizophrenia towards an ultimate, as yet elusive, fact.

Subsequent researchers would propose late-onset schizophrenia as occurring after the age of forty-five and very late-onset schizophrenia as occurring after the age of sixty-five, while reincluding the previously abandoned childhood-onset schizophrenia. Later-onset schizophrenia is generally considered to have the same symptoms as childhood schizophrenia, only more severe.[7] DSM-III-R was a supposed nonsignificant text revision, but a significant population would have been rendered no longer 'immune'.[8]

Schizophrenia is presented, across its different incarnations, as a biological disease. And yet, it's hard to imagine an age limit being suddenly imposed on another medical diagnosis in the same way – say, diabetes. Imagine, for a moment, if all of a sudden, anyone over the age of forty-five with the symptoms of diabetes, couldn't access treatment. We would want to know what change in our understanding of the underlying biology of the condition motivated this redefinition. If there was no clear explanation, the original update would surely be deemed irresponsible, putting people's lives at risk. Somehow, though, psychiatry isn't held to the same standards. Despite the supposedly biological basis of its diseases, we do not receive the same biological explanations, or justifications as medical diagnoses.

In the case of 'schizoaffective disorder', which incorporates people with symptoms associated with both manic depression and schizophrenia, psychiatry solved the issue of the so-called 'nonspecificity' of these symptoms (symptoms that didn't fit into the existing categories) by inventing yet another label. There was no need to discard schizophrenia as a diagnosis when it could no longer contend with the multitude of variations. Instead, the DSM simply sprouted a new disease. The diagnoses of schizophrenia and schizoaffective disorder combined, effectively encompass more or less everyone who shows a psychotic disturbance, apart from a small minority who can be labelled categorically as having bipolar disorder or a discrete drug-induced episode.[9] The term schizophrenia as it is used in psychiatry, in all its forms and subdivisions, seems to hold the same limitless capacity for mopping up meaning as it does in the popular imagination.

The biological hope

While the definitions of schizophrenia have shapeshifted through time, there has been one consistent certainty underpinning them all: dysfunction. As we saw in Chapter 2, in the third edition of the DSM, however, mental disorders were defined as purely biological problems. They were defined by the American Psychiatric Association as 'behavioural, psychological, or biological dysfunction[s]', and not just '[disturbances] in the relationship between the individual and society',[10] laying the foundations for a biological worldview that saw madness as a deficit in individual bodies, rather than responses to a particular context.

Today, the wide-ranging experiences grouped together under the label of schizophrenia are supposedly connected by a common, biological explanation. The American Psychiatric Association describes schizophrenia as a biological 'chronic brain disorder'. Whatever the symptoms are or may have been, we are reassured, the disease exists in the body, in the molecules of hormones and neurotransmitters that determine our moods and behaviours, or the structure of the brain, determined by our DNA. While psychiatrists may still be exploring the range of symptoms associated with the disease, knowing that they are targeting an underlying, biological, disorder assures us that the treatments, at least, are robust. Perhaps we need not worry about the lack of consensus on the definition of this highly medicated disease. Perhaps biological mechanisms explain what the broad, catch-all language of symptoms in the DSM cannot.

From its inception, schizophrenia has always been an open question. Paradoxically, it has also been where psychiatry has purported to know the most. After all, schizophrenia provided the basis on which it first asserted its authority as a new science.

When the German psychiatrist Emil Kraepelin (1856–1926) set out to produce the first classification of discrete mental disorders in 1883, he did so based on observable symptoms. The biological basis of these conditions was not known, so he left this as an open question, fixing his efforts on what he could observe.

Biological hope – the belief that science would eventually catch up with psychiatry and prove the existence of these various disorders beyond the external symptoms displayed – was at the core of the diagnosis for schizophrenia laid down by early practitioners, but biology itself was not at the base of their definitions, and this hope was never realised. When the psychiatrists, sometimes called 'neo-Kraepelinians', took over the task of establishing a modern classification in the 1980 version of the DSM, one that would be rooted firmly in the methods of the medical discipline, they reverted to these same guiding principles, taking an operational approach to classification. They would go by what they knew, and what they knew was not so very different from what the early psychiatrists of the nineteenth century had determined through the lens of eugenic thinking to be sensible categories of behaviour. They would cluster together the symptoms they could observe plain and clear, in lieu of the biological evidence that was, always, 'soon to come'.

We have already seen that through the 1990s and into the new millennium, the biological hope was how a psychiatry rooted in neuroscience gained traction. The promise of the ever-imminent biological explanation also made it close to impossible to prove any study wrong, because the concept was always *just about* to be fleshed out biologically. Schizophrenia and its symptoms were not yet properly known, so if a subclassification was disproven, this didn't undermine the existence of the concept per se, it just meant more scientific work was needed. The existence of an underlying cause for the symptoms was never in question.

And so, psychiatry forged ahead on its biological mission, lost in the dizzying refractions of its biological prism. Almost no organ or brain region had been left unimplicated at one stage or another in the search for the cause of schizophrenia. It has been a colourful, violent and inconclusive history; from the hunt for localised brain damage in the nineteenth century, to the belief that it was a disease resulting from microbial infection of the gut, the teeth, appendices, ovaries, testes, or even the colon (with the accompanying colonic irrigations proposed as a cure) and the practice of cutting out infectious parts of the brain (with predictably fatal consequences for patients) through the twentieth century, to induce a state of so-called calm. Investigations continue to show population-wide and individual variation. There is no common indicator in the brain connecting the wide-ranging experiences associated with schizophrenia.

An ever-growing mass of brain studies continue to report particularities that characterise the brains of people with the diagnosis of schizophrenia. And, at the same time, the causal connection between the two is repeatedly refuted. The evidence shows time and again that the poor long-term outcome for people with schizophrenia has little to do with physical brain problems. Recent studies have found no association between schizophrenia and progressive cognitive decline;[11] the reported cognitive deficits of schizophrenic patients also persist over time, rather than deteriorating as you would expect of a degenerative brain disease. While some schizophrenic patients do experience deterioration in functioning, this more likely reflects poor access, or adherence, to treatment, the effects of concurrent conditions, and, as ever, social isolation, discrimination or financial struggle.

And yet the sheer quantity of biological studies on the genetics and neurology of schizophrenia continue to sustain the hope that a biological explanation is imminent. That the term 'schizophrenia' has persisted through time sustains an illusion of progress. In fact, behind the name, there still exists a multitude of conflicting theoretical positions. The legitimacy of the DSM has amped up the financial stakes for psychiatrists working in North America, where using the DSM entitles them to compensation by insurance companies, FDA approval, and grant funding. As early as 1979, two psychiatrists had already summarised the issue: 'We find the observation that the very existence of schizophrenia grants, conferences and manuals provides considerable reification for a major psychiatric conceptualisation that many believe to be illogically derived.'[12] This circular logic that schizophrenia must exist because a system has built around it persists.

From this perspective, psychiatry's dogged pursuit of a failing method, begins to make sense. Professional credibility, underpinned by financial incentive for pharmaceutical industries, is at stake. From the beginning, psychiatry's legitimacy has depended on the promise that one day it will come good on its biological promise. The concept of 'schizophrenia' has withstood the test of time because psychiatry needs it to. The diagnosis is so woven up with the history and legitimacy of the profession, that you could say that what psychiatrists are really debating when they talk about schizophrenia, is psychiatry itself. This professional insecurity is never addressed but is ever implicit in the increasingly exasperated discussions on schizophrenia in influential medical journals, as some continue to defend the concept against critics who question at the very least whether, given the social, cultural and environmental facts involved, a purely biological concept of schizophrenia is fit for purpose.[13] The tension is palpable as the split widens between psychiatrists who still vest hope in genes and brain scans for solutions, and a growing body of researchers and clinicians who are arguing, ever more ardently, that time is up on an approach that is not helping patients today.

Biological compassion

It is important to recognise the search for biological explanations for mental distress as a choice, and not an inevitability. Amidst today's highly medicalised culture, it is easy to forget that other explanations and forms of support for mental distress are possible. As intuitive as it might be to most of us that the things that happen to us in our lives affect our state of mind, we revert to psychiatric treatment as a default when we feel out of control. But the dominance of the medical psychiatric approach could have been otherwise. Biological psychiatrists have fought hard over the past centuries, and again in recent decades to maintain their status as medical authority on the mind.

The biological view in psychiatry was solidified in the 1980s, as we have seen, in part through the hope of neuroscience, which was also, increasingly, tied to genetics. Studying madness in relation to genetics had become more uncomfortable after the Nazis' eugenics, but by the 1970s, psychiatrists in favour of a biological approach had managed to frame their plight to find a biological origin as the compassionate option. Biological psychiatrists now claimed that they offered a humane alternative to the rival talking therapies. Rather than blaming individuals or their parents for their mental struggles, they saw mental illnesses as diseases like any other.[14] They were nobody's 'fault'. The mentally ill would no longer be stigmatised and deserved the same care as patients with cancer or heart disease.[15]

It is understandable that this approach was preferable to the burden the parents of schizophrenic people carried at this time. Especially in the American context, which had seen a deinstitutionalisation of prisons: the decision of state governments across the country to release large numbers of institutionalised psychiatric patients, many in long-term care, back into the community. The vision was that, with prescriptions of medications that would keep their worst symptoms in check, the schizophrenic patients would be able to receive care on an outpatient basis in community mental health centres, thus saving the state money. The reality was that the care available was poorly organised and insufficient. This meant that, though parents were relieved of the psychological burden of blame for their children's struggles, this was replaced, for many, by the material weight of caregiving responsibilities. It is understandable that many patients and their families continued to place hope with the prospect of a biological 'cure' on the horizon. Yet psychiatrists should never have stood in where social support structures were needed. Governments had left people desperate and susceptible to ungrounded hope, and left families having to fill the void left by unrealised promises and ineffective treatments. Social solutions were needed all along, and, as we'll see, are still where the real hope lies for those suffering mentally, as well as the communities that support them.

The biological psychiatrists of the 1980s spun a narrative that seemed to have at its heart the plight of the patient. Yet in failing to ask whether this approach was delivering on its promise, they were choosing to sustain a profession over people.

The insistence on biology, specifically neurology and genetics, has precluded alternative ways of understanding the experiences psychiatrists have described as schizophrenia. It has, for one, left the social assumptions and consequences contained in the 'biological' diagnosis unquestioned. This has opened up the concept to manipulation – both by the profession and by governments, as they continue to leverage the loose definition to perpetuate harmful ideas about minoritised people that justify societal neglect. The biological focus that remains indifferent to actual evidence in the field of schizophrenia is bad science in both senses of the word – it is non-rigorous and myopic and has delivered few consistent findings, and it is also unethical, leading to bad policies and poor health outcomes, especially among those who already suffer the consequences of social disparities.

The biological score

Enthusiasm for finding a genetic basis for schizophrenia today is as alive as it was in the early days of psychiatry. The pipeline view once again obfuscated the crucial lack of evidence for this supposed brain-based concept. Schizophrenia continues to be one of the best-funded research areas in mental health – in the UK, second only to depression. In academic journals today schizophrenia continues to be variously characterised as 'a debilitating neurological disorder', a 'devastating, highly heritable brain disorder', or a 'brain disorder with predominantly genetic risk factors'.[16]

Despite these claims, though, there is to this day no conclusive evidence that schizophrenia has a neurological cause, nor, as much of the research claims, that it is straightforwardly inherited through genes.[17] As one team of University College London psychiatrists put it in a paper authored in 2015: 'Schizophrenia is a label that implies the presence of a biological disease, but no specific bodily disorder has been demonstrated.'[18] Or, in the following year, a clinical psychologist and professor of health and social policy from the University of Liverpool on the supposed genetic link: There are no 'schizophrenia genes ... molecular genetic research simply does not support the standard "genes for schizophrenia" story.'[19] From the US, a psychiatrist committed to the medical view of schizophrenia: 'NIMH's [The National Institute of Mental Health] genetics investment has yielded almost nothing clinically useful for individuals currently affected.'[20]

Yet still, the genetic research persists.

The psychologist Jay Joseph has dedicated his career to reopening the debates around the heritability of schizophrenia. The foundations of much of this research, he shows, are deeply flawed, to the extent that publications have produced the findings that dog ownership, vegetarianism and concern for nature are only fractionally less heritable than schizophrenia.[21] The foundations of much of the genetic research we take as the forefront of some of the most hopeful science for human health today, glaringly needs revisiting.

Previously, researchers had set their sights on finding a 'candidate gene' for schizophrenia – suspect genes based on their location on a chromosome or their known role in other functions. The hunt for the candidate gene, however, has since been recognised across the literature as a failed pursuit.[22] Researchers have since turned to genome-wide association studies (GWAS) to build more intricate theories about the genetic origins of schizophrenia. Introduced in 2005, GWAS detects associations, or correlations, between genetic variants and traits in samples from populations. Using samples of tens of thousands of patients and controls, many genes, each with a microscopic effect, have been linked to schizophrenia. These genes are then assimilated to produce a 'polygenic risk score', which describes a person's total genetic risk. A risk score gives the impression of a measurable, predictable outcome based on biology, but the certainty ascribed to genes in predicting schizophrenia continues to be misleading.

Some psychiatrists are working to temper genetic enthusiasm and build a more realistic picture of their predictive power in mental health. One study drew on data from a Dutch mental health survey to show how the contribution of genetic risk tends to be 'evaluated on the basis of statistical significance-testing in massive samples, in which minute effects acquire statistical significance', but may be *clinically* meaningless – in other words, these associations do not help predict who will actually have the experiences associated with schizophrenia.[23] They found that social-environmental circumstances, particularly childhood trauma and perceived status gap, drive 99.5 per cent of a person's likelihood to develop the symptoms associated with schizophrenia. Genetic factors explain only about 0.5 per cent. This echoes previous research that has also shown that, even after sequencing the entire genome, genetic factors only explained 2.28 per cent of whether a person received a diagnosis of schizophrenia.[24]

The hunt for genetic predictors of mental suffering omits a 'factor' that is actually the prerequisite for any meaningful interpretation of genetic information: the environment.

Without understanding the role that environmental triggers play, these supposed genetic findings, so prolific in the research on schizophrenia (and mental disease generally), show us a vague correlation between genes and a hypothetical disease that tells us nothing about this relationship; we don't know whether they are causally related – whether the genes in some way cause the disease, or whether there are other factors at play. While geneticists may acknowledge, if you ask them, that their research only offers part of a much bigger picture, the funding and hype around genetic studies easily misconstrues and overvalues their contribution, at the cost of other, crucial, parts of the picture. This misguided enthusiasm has fuelled the field in its concerted effort to prove, using the authoritative language of genetics, the existence of a disease that is already assumed to exist.

One polygenic risk score study,[25] published in the science journal *Nature* in 2016, showed how the genetic variations found to be more present in those diagnosed with 'schizophrenia' also happen to be involved in immune function. These genetic variations – C4 proteins – trigger inflammation in response to injury or infection. Inflammation is supposed to protect the body. It makes sense, then, that abnormalities in C4 proteins are associated with autoimmune diseases, such as lupus and kidney disease.[26] But an inflammatory immune response has also been associated with people diagnosed with schizophrenia[27] and the discovery of higher immune cell activity in the brains of those considered to be at risk of schizophrenia has also led to the suggestion that early anti-inflammatory treatments might provide effective treatment.[28]

These findings may be promising, and they may indeed provide useful biological interventions. They could even help explain why genes associated with immune function may be different for people with schizophrenia. However, this continues just to be a correlation. Connecting these biological findings builds a more detailed picture of what happens but they still don't explain how changes in C4 proteins or immune responses might cause schizophrenia in the first place. This research doesn't offer more than another theory of what that mechanism might be. It may be true that genes involved in immune response have an effect on the brain that causes the psychotic symptoms currently associated with schizophrenia. But it is also possible that the increased activity of C4 proteins are the *result* and not the cause of a chain of events in a person's life.

The problem with the highly prevalent genetic studies is not only what they do or do not find, but also what they omit: the social context that drives us into distress. Scientific investigations rely on a reaching into the unknown – sometimes they fail, sometimes they deliver. But by failing to consider the context in which distress arises, scientists have misrepresented the question that needs answering. They have whittled the *experience* of distress into a hunt for a causal gene. Even if we found that a gene was related to a mental experience, we would still not understand *how* that gene creates the experiences associated with schizophrenia. Genes, like bodies and minds, cannot be understood in a vacuum. This makes sense when we consider that we have genes in order to allow us to adapt to our environments. It is not the gene itself, but its interaction with an environment to produce a trait that we are talking about when we talk about genes. Genes are the product of a dialogue with our surroundings and only make sense from this dynamic perspective. A gene does not exist without a body to work on, or through. No gene will have an effect if it is not activated or deactivated in the body, and that happens as a result of environmental triggers. Sometimes, changing environmental factors such as pollution, or viruses, or psychological trauma, might cause a change to the expression of the genes, switching them on or off. Sometimes, these changes are passed on to the next generation. But in any case, to speak of genetic variations without an understanding of how these are activated or deactivated, tells us very little about whatever it is we're looking at. It is an observation, not an explanation, or even a very adequate description of a process. And we need to remember this, when we read accounts of breakthrough genetic explanations of mental disease.

One helpful case in point for the role of biology in psychosis and its relationship to trauma comes from studies on postpartum psychosis. I spoke to the professor of neurobiology of psychosis at King's College London, Paola Dazzan, who now works clinically as a perinatal psychiatrist, but who started her career working on a project investigating the higher prevalence of schizophrenia among minoritised groups. She was a biological psychiatrist and so was made responsible for the biological aspects of their study, while her colleague focused on the social causes. The work they did, she says, has informed everything she has done since, and describes herself as 'a biological psychiatrist who is always looking at the body in relation to a certain environment'. Professor Dazzan is adamant that biology cannot be understood out of context. This is powerfully demonstrated in her more recent work on postpartum psychosis, one of the most severe perinatal mental health conditions she works with. This is a useful case of psychosis for psychiatrists wanting to parse out the role of biology, as it is a clearly delineated biological event that starts after delivery.

'This form of psychosis,' Professor Dazzan explains, 'usually arises within two weeks of giving birth, so clearly there is an association between this big biological event, where women give birth, oestrogen levels decrease dramatically, cortisol levels go down dramatically, and very suddenly they develop these psychotic symptoms.' Yet while investigating women who experience psychosis following childbirth has helped elucidate the biological onset,[29] it has, at the same time, revealed the limitations of biological explanations: 'Of course, not all women who give birth experience postpartum psychosis. There are so many environmental factors at play.' In other studies, Professor Dazzan and her colleagues showed that women who experience postpartum psychosis are more likely to have experienced trauma or abuse, making these experiences key to understanding how the biological mechanisms relating to postpartum psychosis are triggered in the first place.[30] She added: 'Biology can never explain it all, because biology is mostly a consequence of what we have in our environment.'

It is more common, today, to see research on the so-called social determinants of mental health under the bracket of what is often called the 'bio-psycho-social' approach. Here social factors, socioeconomic status, education or job-related stresses, might be included in explanations of mental disorder, but these often include environmental factors that simply protect or provoke a problem that exists separately, in the brain; the environment isn't separable from our brain, and is intricately connected to the brain throughout our lives. This is not to say that people don't vary biologically, it is contesting the primacy of biology in explanations and solutions to mental distress. Environmental issues are always part of the picture, and also more immediately tractable than many of the biological factors that currently take up the bulk of research and funding.

The biological origin stories of schizophrenia, whether focused on brains or genes, or, indeed, hormones, do not explain causation; they offer an inoperable correlation that makes no sense without an understanding of the environment in which they operate. Stripped of the context to which people respond, their experiences become anomalous aberrations, rather than meaningful reactions. Experiences like psychosis can only be understood as meaningful in relation to the things that happen to someone, and they can easily be understood as dysfunction when they are robbed of the context that makes them meaningful. A purely biological lens all too easily directs shame and blame towards the individual and away from the social world that fosters unbearable conditions for so many people's minds. That social world, though, is where we'll find the most devastating causes of mental disease, and also the most effective responses.

Research that places the genetic observations like the ones described in an environmental context are beginning to suggest how biological factors might reflect, rather than cause, the psychological distress called schizophrenia in the genetic studies. Genes register these effects, but they do not cause them.

One such environmental factor shown to have a direct impact on the expression of C_4, is childhood trauma. A 2007 study linked higher levels of a protein that regulates the C_4 immune system with childhood adversity.[31] This effect was measured even twenty years after the period of trauma. The effects of childhood trauma on immune response have similarly been shown in adults with auto-immune diseases such as rheumatoid arthritis[32] and chronic fatigue syndrome,[33] so this finding could contribute to a growing picture. The point, then, is not that biology is irrelevant when it comes to understanding psychiatric conditions, but instead that biology tells us nothing when it is the only thing considered. It is possible that psychoses are similarly the result of autoimmune disorder, triggered by childhood trauma, including bullying, emotional, sexual and physical abuse, incest, neglect, parental loss, and the stress of immigration, urbanicity, poverty, relative poverty and social marginalisation.[34]

Once we understand the role of the environment in triggering these biological responses, we open up the possibility of addressing the actual source of the problem in people's lives. Biology can never offer us a full picture of how we become distressed. We will always need to understand the world that makes us so.

A non-biological death sentence

While the link between trauma and psychotic disorders in the field of genetics barely registers in the wider social consciousness, it is in fact, relatively well known in other areas of psychiatry and psychology. Around the same time that the studies on 'breakthrough' genetic links to schizophrenia were hitting the news, one study, for example, showed a connection between childhood adversity, particularly sexual abuse, and delusions and hallucinations.[35] Other studies have shown that the greater the number of adverse experiences and/or the higher the severity, the greater the risk of psychosis in adulthood.[36] Those who have experienced constant childhood abuse are almost 50 times more likely to develop psychosis as an adult.[37] As the authors of one of the studies wrote: 'Experiencing multiple childhood traumas appears to give approximately the same risk of developing psychosis as smoking does for developing lung cancer.'[38]

When we follow schizophrenia into the world, we find that, while there are no definitive genetic associations, the symptoms associated with schizophrenia map irrefutably onto the inequalities in societies. Psychosis, it turns out, is more common, with a poorer prognosis and outcome among those who are the primary recipients of trauma in our world. In high-income countries, the occurrence of psychotic disorders across all minoritised ethnic populations combined is between 1.5 and 3 times higher than the rest of the population.[39] In the UK, rates are highest among Black people, between 4 and 6 times higher relative to the rest of the population.[40] Yet in other countries, like the Netherlands, rates are especially high for Moroccan and Surinamese populations, but less so for Turkish.[41] It isn't entirely clear why this is, but other studies have shown elevated levels of perceived discrimination for Surinamese and Moroccan people compared to Turkish people with psychosis, and have suggested that the associated stress may help explain differences in migrant experiences affecting rates of psychosis.[42] Turkish people in these studies reported a greater sense of social cohesion. Lead author of the study, Professor Jean-Paul Selten, recalled how at the time of the study, Turkish young men admitted for psychosis would more often be accompanied by family members to support and advocate for them. This sense of social cohesion has decreased in the second generation, where rates of psychosis have sadly increased for the Turkish population.[43]

Another study conducted in East London showed differences within migrant groups. The boroughs included in this particular research were Hackney, Newham and Tower Hamlets. The data for the study was collected between 1996 and 2000, long before the 2012 Olympics led to some substantial neighbourhood regeneration of the area, and long before large parts of Hackney, and parts of the other two boroughs, underwent gentrification and became a beloved of hipsters and influencers. At the time, these boroughs were some of the most deprived in England, and the UK, and had some of the highest proportions of non-White and migrant groups. In particular, these neighbourhoods were, and are, home to very high proportions of people from Bangladeshi and Pakistani backgrounds – both first generation migrants and British-born descendants. This is still the case today despite the gentrification. The researchers found that rates of psychotic disorders among those from Pakistan and Bangladesh in these areas were particularly high among women compared to men, also raising questions about the additional social stresses women face.[44]

What is not included in the paper, the lead researcher and professor in epidemiology in psychiatry Jeremy Coid told me, is that a disproportionate number of people experiencing their first episode of psychosis in the borough of Newham were asylum seekers or refugees. At that time, Newham had the cheapest accommodation in London. Other boroughs had paid to house their refugees on the other side of the city. The results showing higher rates of psychosis in these boroughs generally reflect these social trends and population shifts. Another Swedish study has similarly found that incidence of psychotic disorders was especially high among refugees relative to other migrants.[45] These results point to the role that stress and trauma must play in the onset of psychosis: refugees, and asylum seekers, are already fleeing war, natural disaster, or prosecution. They then face the difficulties of marginalisation and discrimination other migrants do, but with greater insecurity and the fear of exportation looming over them. Other studies confirm that the environment matters when it comes to psychosis. One study of psychosis in urban and rural sites across five European countries showed that the comparative risks of minoritised groups varied depending on setting; the particular stresses of an environment determined the rates of psychosis, even among those already connected by the experience of discrimination and poverty.[46]

These various findings point to complex multifactorial explanations for increased prevalence among some subpopulations compared to others, but they are consistent in showing that the distinctive experiences of dislocation, and the particular social context and the social positions groups of people hold, help to explain the prevalence of an experience that so many scientists still claim to be caused by heritable brain dysfunction. The experiences described as schizophrenia have repeatedly been connected to stress and trauma. We need to invest much more into understanding the social dynamics that make people psychotic, whatever their genes.

I spoke to Professor Craig Morgan, an epidemiologist at King's College London, about the studies he conducted alongside Professor Dazzan, published in 2006, that showed a higher prevalence of 'schizophrenia' among African Caribbean and later the Black African communities in South London, parts of Nottingham, and Bristol.[47] [48] In his work, Professor Morgan is particularly interested in how rates of distress vary across populations. The study involved about 500 people with psychoses, and a similar number without psychoses as a comparison group. They also followed up with everyone over time, documenting the course and outcome of their psychoses ten years on. The study was set up, Morgan explained, to investigate what was at that time a frequently reported finding that there were higher rates of psychoses among minority ethnic groups in the UK, specifically among the African Caribbean, and since then Black African population. If there was a disparity, Morgan and his colleagues also wanted to understand why. They produced clear evidence that there were marked disparities between ethnic groups, findings that have been replicated in subsequent studies across different contexts.[49]

At the time, this finding was somewhat controversial. The study contributed to an ongoing debate in the field, also reported on in the newspapers,[50] which asked whether the disparities observed between groups were real, or merely the result of researcher's bias; in this case, that psychiatrists were more inclined to diagnose schizophrenia when dealing with Black males in particular – problematic, as was rightly noted, given that Black men were also more likely to be subjected to compulsory detentions and police involvement in admissions. This tension runs through studies showing racial and gender bias in psychosis.

The earliest reports on disparities in schizophrenia among minoritised communities in the UK were conducted in the late 1970s and early 1980s. At this time, to link ethnicity or race with an increased risk of a heavily stigmatised disorder that was considered to be primarily genetic, came uncomfortably close to racist ideologies peddled historically by the Nazis and white supremacists. And indeed, population differences in genetic risk, obstetric complications or viral infections were proposed, fuelling initial concerns about the links being drawn between race, ethnicity, biological deficits and schizophrenia.[51] Considered from this perspective, the over-diagnosis of schizophrenia here stemmed from wider stereotypes which were forcefully refracted through the lens of psychiatry, and used as a basis for societal neglect and oppression.[52]

Schizophrenia has historically been constructed as a Black disease. Links to stress and trauma in inducing the state of psychosis associated with schizophrenia helps to explain higher rates among Black people. But it is also important to understand that the characteristics and behaviours associated with this diagnostic category were shaped by eugenic thinking in the first place, which has long tied schizophrenia to ideas about Black biological inferiority.[53] Brain-based explanations served to further entrench preconceived racial stereotypes.

As journalist and author Micha Frazer-Carroll shows in her book *Mad World*, psychiatrists developing the earliest definitions of schizophrenia were guided by eugenic ideas that associated the disease with Black 'degeneracy' and 'primitiveness'.[54] The British colonial psychiatrist H. L. Gordon, who worked in a Kenyan mental hospital in the 1930s asserted, in the language of the cutting-edge brain science of the time, that African people developed the disorder due to the 'inferior durability' of their brain cells.[55]

In the 1960s, the disease was again, only slightly more subtly, racialised when US psychiatrists Walter Bromberg and Franck Simon suggested that Malcolm X and the civil rights movement had sparked a wave of violent schizophrenic symptoms and paranoid 'racial antagonism' in African Americans. As more Black people joined the movement and consciously dissented against the racist societal order, Bromberg and Simon dubbed this phenomenon 'the protest psychosis'.[56] The psychiatric diagnosis fed into an idea that these people were not in a state of mind to be taken seriously, not deserving of their straightforward demands for fair and equal treatment.

When the second edition of the DSM was released in 1968, the diagnostic criteria described schizophrenia as making people 'hostile' and 'aggressive'[57] – attributes that, Frazer-Carroll points out, overlap with stereotypes of Black violence and criminality, and during this period, Black people in the US and Britain were increasingly diagnosed with schizophrenia. These historic associations between Black stereotypes and schizophrenia are reflected in the especially high rates of diagnosis that persist among Black men today, who are 10 times more likely to receive a diagnosis of a psychotic disorder than White men.[58] When we look at the rates of psychosis associated with schizophrenia, we need to think not only about the social causes of experiences associated with the medical diagnosis, but also about how the category is constructed in relation to prejudice and inequity. This is how an exclusively medical perspective on mental distress obscures and reinforces discrimination and obfuscates the evidence that might bolster the argument for social support.

Critics in the 1970s and 80s argued that the distress arising from difficult conditions and life experiences continued to be systematically misdiagnosed as schizophrenia in minority groups. It continues to be true that the weight of a history of prejudice encoded in diagnoses and a lack of a methodology that takes account of researcher's biases in interpreting behaviour makes it difficult to distinguish between the effects of the environment on behaviour and the ideas associated with groups of people that researchers project onto them. And in the early 2000s, too, Professor Morgan told me, this wasn't helped by the diagnostic labels that epidemiologists, who generally study diseases in populations, were still required to use. At the time, he explained, funding bodies were driven by a disorder model, and so geared towards finding the causes of a specific disorder like schizophrenia. This model has frequently led psychiatrists to a confirmation bias in which they have searched for biological evidence in order to affirm their views – and to secure more funding. As far as Morgan is concerned, concepts like schizophrenia have a limited time left, and are not that useful in any case: they 'don't capture much about the differences between people and experiences.'

That is why, in academic research like Morgan's, there has been a gradual shift away from diagnostic terms like 'schizophrenia' since he conducted the study, towards a view based on dimensions of distress – a view that sees symptoms like psychosis as just one possible expression of a state of distress that we all experience in different ways and to different degrees, depending on our environments and the things that happen to us. It is easier to make sense of the disparities in mental and emotional distress when, rather than treating these as biological diseases that exist in people, we view these differences in relation to their environments, across communities. Take that perspective, and the question becomes: 'Are there higher levels of severe emotional distress among some populations relative to others?' The answer is obviously 'yes'. This is intuitive, Professor Morgan said: 'We know from our own personal lives that if difficult and challenging things happen, it increases our emotional distress – feelings of sadness and anxiety.' On that level it is obvious that there is a clear link between how and where we live our lives and the things that happen to us and our emotional state. 'I don't think this should be controversial,' Morgan said.

Research today continues to show how psychosis is related to a range of social risk factors, such as exposure to impoverished and urban environments, migration, recent adverse experiences in adulthood, as well as childhood trauma.[59] From this perspective, it is easier not only to make sense of the quantitative differences in distress between populations, but also the shape their distress takes. As Morgan explained:

Being in contexts where there's high levels of threat and uncertainty, all of those things come together to create a context where people feel like they're being singled out by others, they're being persecuted, and that they're being discriminated against. And that is true for many people. In contexts like that, along with poverty and high levels of isolation, it is not difficult to imagine how that kind of experience might generalise to feeling that lots of people are against you, or the whole world is against you, and that then it becomes more systematising to believe that the state is against you, that the state apparatus is against you, CIA or MI5 is spying on you. So there's a direct link between the types of experiences people have and the emotional distress and the form it takes.

Research like Morgan's puts individuals previously diagnosed on an individual basis (based on an underlying assumption of the shared biological pathology of an imagined diagnostic group) back into the world, to understand what the patterns in populations tell us about how individual people respond to adversity.

There is now a broad consensus in epidemiological research that increased rates of psychosis in minoritised groups are a consequence of external environmental factors, in particular related to social conditions, position and experience across the life course. Slowly, recognition is growing that the epidemiological perspective is one that shows us much more about mental distress than the prism of medical illness. Mental distress maps seamlessly onto social inequality because it reflects what happens to us. This is the real sense in which the individual mind is a barometer for societal distress. And so we must begin to question whether we can meaningfully discuss schizophrenia as an individual rather than social disease at all.

This view aligns with non-biological research being conducted into how states of psychosis emerge. The psychiatrist Jim van Os, who is a significant force in trying to reform the field of schizophrenia and psychiatry as a whole, shows how rather than a biological causation, it is possible to deduce an *emotional* chain of causation for psychosis. Non-psychotic states like irritability can lead to anxiety, then depression, and psychosis.[60] As environmental conditions exacerbate these emotions, individuals can tip into a more severe state of distress. From this perspective, we all have the potential for – and in fact, many of us do experience – psychotic symptoms to various degrees.[61] Only, for those exposed to accumulating environmental triggers, and experiencing a greater range of mental distress, lasting psychotic symptoms becomes more likely. Which makes a diagnosis, according to the DSM, more likely.

This emotional rather than biological view of psychotic risk, has proven much more effective in identifying who needs help.[62] Focusing on non-psychotic risk factors are better predictors of psychosis, rather than any static 'biomarkers' of a discrete disease that scientists have found. This view, again, frames mental distress as a response to a social and physical environment. Van Os goes so far as to define psychosis as 'the human capacity, served by thousands of genetic variants, to see meaning in environmental noise.' The state of psychosis associated with schizophrenia reflects a universal human tendency to make meaning of our environments. This is not explained by genes or biology, as much as these may play a role. Echoing Morgan's statement above, Van Os says that individual variation in how we make sense of the things that happen to us needs to be understood by looking at the environments we live in, and that human responses to their environments are survival strategies, rather than symptoms of inherent brokenness.

When we experience persistent threats in our surroundings, we may begin to perceive danger when it is no longer there. This is all so intuitive when we think about how our feelings and behaviour change through our lives, and yet it is an open question as to how long it will take governments and mental healthcare systems to embrace this view. Take stock of the research to date, and most will agree that there is a more hopeful alternative to the biological dreams of a system of historically loaded diagnoses ever awaiting biological confirmation. The fact is that there is no evidence to suggest that biological variations, like genetic or neurodevelopmental differences, can explain the high rates of psychotic disorders in minoritised populations. There is ample evidence, on the other hand, that environmental triggers, experiences and social context, interact and act on the body over time, to increase the risk of psychoses. And that evidence shows us that psychosis occurs most where the environments people live in are hostile.

Taking this view, levels of mental distress become an effective barometer for the functioning of society. The higher the levels of distress in individuals, the greater the challenges we're facing as a society. This also points the finger at the root of the problem, which, while it may involve biology, is predominantly societal and will require societal change. The symptoms of schizophrenia currently significantly reduce the lifespan of those who suffer – life expectancy of someone with psychosis is reduced by about a fifth compared to the average[63] – and this is predominantly due to inadequate social infrastructure and care.[64] Through and through, our understanding of the disorder we still call 'schizophrenia' is the result of a grave form of social inequality. Many people with psychoses are not receiving the right care, due to an insistence on biological cure that has repeatedly proven ineffective. More so, by insisting on this biological view, we have neglected the societal changes needed to support those who are most susceptible to psychoses in the first place. Mental distress will only further entrench existing social disparities, as they further disadvantage individuals in society.

Psychosis is a social problem and needs social solutions.

Research that takes this social view has yielded more workable findings than two centuries' worth of biological studies. It's time we start taking the recommendations of those researchers seriously.

The hope in discontent

Professor van Os has never left any doubt about his stance on the biological concept of schizophrenia. He has taken a brazen approach to fighting the field's dogmas. He first entered the debate around the term with a research paper published in the *British Medical Journal* in 1993 titled 'Schizophrenia sans frontieres: concepts of schizophrenia among French and British psychiatrists'.[65] In it, he and his colleagues described how the concept of schizophrenia in France was entirely different from that in the UK. 'They differed in terms of symptoms, demography, treatment and prognosis,' he told me. French psychiatrists reserved the diagnosis for people with an onset before the age of forty-five, for whom the disease was chronic, and showed little sign of improving. In the UK, clinicians included patients with a 'good' (defined medically, in terms of recovery from the symptoms of the perceived disease) outcome and late onset. French psychiatrists referred to concepts from psychoanalysis to explain the disease and gave much greater importance to family dynamics and parental factors than their British counterparts. The UK psychiatrists preferred neurodevelopmental and genetic explanations over social ones. UK psychiatrists also diagnosed schizophrenia in people experiencing delusions, while the French didn't. There were striking differences over the role of family dynamics and parental factors in the causation of schizophrenia; French psychiatrists gave these much more importance than their British colleagues. 'Yet, in both countries there was a group of people called "psychiatrists",' van Os went on, 'who were completely convinced that they knew what schizophrenia was.' Even two decades after the paper's publication, van Os still described these findings with an air of disbelief. This investigation made him understandably sceptical of the validity of the term, and also, more generally, of the kind of knowledge held by psychiatrists.

In 2015, van Os made a real splash on the scene with an opinion piece co-authored with Dutch scientists, patients and their relatives and published in a national newspaper, titled 'Schizophrenia does not exist.'[66] In it, they urged the psychiatric community to drop what they called the 'contested' term 'schizophrenia'. The diagnosis had existed since the birth of psychiatry, but it had to go. Their reasoning was multiple. For one, the term implied a bleak prognosis; its inherent and chronic nature suggested that recovery was unlikely. From their experience of working with patients with symptoms associated with schizophrenia, this simply was not the case. In fact, they write, only 20 per cent of people who experience psychosis will not recover, most do or learn to manage their symptoms and return to their regular lives. About a third of people diagnosed with schizophrenia experience complete remission of symptoms, and the rest are able to work and live independently.[67] Their second main gripe was that the biological experiences remained inconclusive: 'Sixty years of intense biological research has yielded neither solid nor clinically relevant biology-based distinctions.'[68] Most distressingly, though, they argued, it wasn't clear what biology has to do with the actual experience of patients. As van Os has written elsewhere: 'It remains unknown if, how and to what degree mental phenomena are represented physically and – even if this were so – why this would be relevant to understanding mental suffering.'[69] The term was inaccurate, uninformative, and, given this state of affairs, outright irresponsible.

When van Os made his first claims about the need for a different approach in psychiatry, he was met with resistance. 'There was a big national newspaper article, written by my colleagues, published in 2015, saying I was an "anti-psychiatrist".' Van Os laughed as he recounted the story. 'That was my own fault, of course. When you go in with a firm stance like that, shaking things up, you're inviting criticism. But that was good.' He tells the story with a light-heartedness that isn't flippant, but with a sense that disagreement isn't the worst that can happen; with a sense that perhaps the real tragedy lies in the lives neglected in the current mental healthcare system, and not the egos bruised.

After van Os fell out of favour with his colleagues, he started two websites under that same provocative title that headed the eponymous newspaper article, 'Schizophrenia Does Not Exist.'[70] On the website, he reiterated their stance: that there was no scientific proof for this vague association of biology and symptoms as a disease. The website was met with the inevitable wave of critique from the psychiatric community. At the same time, though, it became very popular with people experiencing psychosis. That is because the website was not just a pawn in a professional showdown, but was intended as a tool for people to use; it provided useful information – practical advice for people on how to cope with psychosis in the context of their lives.

'Now we have 1.5 million users every year, and it's well recognised,' he told me. The website became a fixture in the mental health landscape simply because it worked. The proof was in the pudding – people were using it. Its sheer popularity pointed to the void left by psychiatric services, but it also trialled a different approach, focused less on explaining the biological causes of disease, where psychiatrists had made no headway, and more on interventions that seemed to work.

With an undeniable success, van Os was, as he calls it, 'rehabilitated', redeemed by the psychiatric community; just as he had hoped, people came around, eventually. And perhaps with psychiatrists exemplifying the kind of moral compass and ethical resilience van Os did, we can hope that others, too, will risk professional upset in the future – because defensiveness has led the field to stagnation.

As far as schizophrenia itself goes, van Os thinks, things are changing, not just in the Netherlands, but worldwide. At the time of writing, the International Schizophrenia Research Society in Toronto is about to present him with a lifetime achievement award – testament to the fact, he says, that the DSM-based, biomedical approach is on its way out. He was also, tellingly, approached by the University of Utrecht Medical Centre to serve as their new Chair of the Division of Neuroscience – not despite, but *because* of his public health approach.

Of course, reform within psychiatry isn't the only option. To move away from the stigmatising bind of diagnosis, some might choose to abandon psychiatry altogether. The radical survivor movement has long offered alternatives to the medical approach in order to provide a more welcoming home for those struggling with the experiences. The Hearing Voices Network, for example, contests the validity of diagnoses like 'schizophrenia' altogether, and opts firmly for individual, social, spiritual and political explanations of distress.[71] They do not use the language of disease, do not discuss the phenomena of hearing voices or seeing visions as mental illnesses, but instead as experiences that can be understood in relation to a life. The charity helps people access resources that enables them to manage distressing, confusing, or difficult voices or visions. Some of these resources encourage people to manage these experiences by cultivating a compassionate and even positive relationship to them. Their aim is to destigmatise voice-hearing and related experiences in healthcare settings and wider society.

There are many useful personal testimonies on the Hearing Voices Network website that offer a clear idea of what this non-medical approach to managing voices might look like. While there is no singular experience, and every account shows just how intricately these voices are tied up with the fabric of an individual's life and personality, there are some consistencies. First, most reflect a profoundly unhelpful and damaging relationship to their medical prescriptions for the symptoms they were experiencing, not just due to the often-debilitating reactions to incredibly strong tranquiliser medications, but, more importantly, on the grounds that these suppressed the voices they were hearing, hereby contributing to a fearful relationship to them. The stories also show powerfully how, often, once individuals turned their attention to managing their relationship to the voices, they were able to understand how, in most cases, these resembled a response to prior traumatic experiences. In this way, the voices became less threatening, and, in some cases, even provided a useful guide to their feelings. Managing the relationship to their voices, in all cases, has a profoundly transformative effect, empowering them to negotiate a relationship to what was previously a frightening change to their inner world, rather than suppressing symptoms that point to often neglected and meaningful parts of a lived experience and present reality.

Many of the most ambitious visions of a better mental healthcare system see a place for non-medical approaches like these, rooted in survivor movements, alongside the limited use of drugs for people in crisis. The epidemiological research on psychosis, after all, shows the indisputable role of social factors in causing mental distress. If we based our mental healthcare system on this understanding, rather than medical diagnosis, it would look very different. Care would have to address the social determinants of mental distress, like poverty, violence and isolation. It would require a coordinated effort between different services, many non-medical, to meet people's needs, and would need to be properly funded.

It is worth repeating that, of course, the drugs prescribed for schizophrenia patients undoubtedly help some. These antipsychotic drugs, also known as neuroleptic drugs or major tranquillisers, are far from ideal. They are strong mind-altering substances, with side effects that can range from skin problems to seizures and neurological disorders.[72] Every individual will respond differently, and their reaction is unpredictable, so doctors administer these drugs with a trial-and-error approach. Nonetheless, medication allows some patients to manage severe and frightening experiences and improve the quality of their lives. But we do need to be realistic about the curative power we attribute to these drugs. As we have seen, they are not the cures they are often presented to be, and administering them does not always reflect an understanding of the cause of distress for an individual. Drugs may ameliorate some symptoms for a while (albeit, often, as we have seen, at a great long-term cost to other aspects of their health), but they do not target the neurobiology of a specific disease, as we are often made to believe. The more we overestimate their power, the less incentivised we will be as a society to pursue other potentially far more beneficial treatments, or to investigate and tackle the widespread social issues that continue to perpetuate psychosis in the population, or to consider support that suggests voices and visions might not be inherently problematic at all.

New explanations and coping strategies emerge when the symptoms clumped together into a disease are treated instead as experiences, rather than fear-inducing abnormalities to be suppressed and hidden away. When we allow them to stand as the signposts in a landscape that connects individuals to the world they have to navigate, a world that changes us all every day, and sometimes in more profound, shocking, but nonetheless meaningful ways. We have to allow people the integrity of finding their own meanings in their mental and emotional experiences. It is this understanding that allows anyone to reconcile themselves with the changes in their minds, to form a new relationship to them, and to heal the splits that the world enacts on them. With or without psychiatry, we need to find new models to facilitate the process of individual meaning-making, rather than imposing (medical) definitions; it is the only humane and, to date, the only effective response to mental distress.

Questions, not answers

While the history and present of schizophrenia remains contested, taken in sum, the result is pretty clear. Today, you'll be hard-pressed to find anyone knowledgeable who believes that the biological hunt for schizophrenia's cause has delivered on its scientific or therapeutic promises. As one former director of the US's National Institute of Mental Health put it in 2013: because psychiatry has had no good new ideas about molecular targets for diagnoses and treatments since the 1950s, 'the underlying science remains immature and ... therapeutic development in psychiatry is simply too difficult and too risky.'[73]

The biological hope is dead. As science historian Anne Harrington puts it: 'It is now increasingly clear that biological psychiatry has overreached, overpromised, over-diagnosed, overmedicated, and compromised its principles.'[74] Insisting on biology has meant denying social responsibility. The best treatment for people suffering from symptoms related to schizophrenia has emerged from an understanding of biology in context, and from turning to the social world that exposes some people to mental disease over others. This is a sobering insight into the structural forms of violence societies have condoned over time. But it is also a source of hope. While schizophrenia is one of the most contested diagnoses in psychiatry, it has also been the source of the most innovative new models for thinking about how we treat mental disease. Tackling schizophrenia has been a springboard for thinking about a more widespread shift away from biological reductionism, and towards a system that actually helps. After all, in the words of Jim van Os and his colleagues, 'Schizophrenia doesn't exist, but psychosis does.'

Some would do away even with this concept, as it

problematises an individual experience that is not necessarily distressing to them. In any case, though, psychosis touches on the sense that voice-hearing isn't an elusive biological horizon, but a responsive state of being. These concepts come closer to connecting us all in the propensity for emotional distress. They describe an experience that we can understand to learn about what has happened to a person, rather than what is wrong with them. Terms like 'psychosis' or the non-psychiatric words like 'visions' or 'voices', are practical and actionable. They orient us from the hope and promise of future understanding to the urgent need for intervention, because they name the reality someone is dealing with in the here and now.

Schizophrenia has long been psychiatry's proxy for an answer. Psychiatry, since it birthed schizophrenia, has been preoccupied with answers. That is what we have come to expect of the profession because that is what it purported to offer. But answers are only as good as the questions we ask. The question preoccupying psychiatry over the past centuries has been, 'What is the biological cause of schizophrenia?' The better, more pressing question now seems to me to be: 'How can psychiatry support people experiencing states of psychosis?' And, by extension, how can psychiatry support people in mental distress? When we don't prioritise these questions, people may start looking for alternatives to medical treatment that may do more harm than good.

7

New Frontiers: Psychedelics

On Wednesday 4 September 2019, Johns Hopkins Medicine announced that it was starting a new centre to study psychedelic drugs for mental disorders. The time was ripe for psychedelics to enter psychiatry, and the $17 million centre was reported to be a milestone in a decades-long struggle by 'outsiders' to medicine to have psychedelics taken seriously in science. They had to do something, the research proponents argued, given that the search for new miracle drugs targeting specific regions of the brain seemed to have stagnated, and the turn to psychedelics provided an exciting, alternative route to what was clearly a dead-end solution to mental suffering.[1]

There is a real buzz around the potential of psychedelics in psychiatry. These perception-altering drugs, largely illegal for decades, are now being considered as therapies for a range of mental disorders. Talk abounds of eradicating previously intractable conditions, like OCD, PTSD, chronic anxiety, treatment-resistant depression, alcoholism and eating disorders.[2] We don't need much encouragement, of course – we're primed to hedge our bets on miracle cures, after all; how else to explain a decades-long obsession with medicalised psychiatric cures. Psychedelics may have existed on the margins of psychiatry, but the possibility of 'curing' conditions with a new miracle substance is a familiar script to us all.

The wealthy donors and health non-profits backing the centre, mainly billionaires (many without prior experience in pharmaceuticals, let alone psychedelics), proselytised about the curative hope of their new ventures. Steven Cohen of the Steven & Alexandra Cohen Foundation which funded half of the John Hopkins centre, announced his support in the *New York Times*: 'I strongly believe that we must dare to change the minds of those who think this drug is for recreational purposes only and acknowledge that it is a miracle for many who are desperate for relief from their symptoms or for the ability to cope with their illnesses. It may even save lives.'[3] Cohen's speech is not dissimilar from NIH director Elias Zerhouni's statements about the hope for human health contained in the psychiatric pipeline. New 'remarkable scientific innovations' had the potential to 'be truly transforming for human health,'[4] he wrote in 2005.

This is the same framing of mental experiences as illnesses in order to garner public, financial and political support for psychedelic research. A slew of studies showing the potential for psychedelics in cancer treatment had already set the stage,[5] providing flickers of that same effort to gain scientific traction we have seen across the 'mainstream' pharmaceutical industry. And indeed, the psychedelic industry has already fallen prey to the same industry tactics we saw in the history of marketing antidepressants – developing but also repurposing drugs for new conditions, educating clinician spokespeople, and ramping up media advertising.[6] The hype in media coverage and the seduction of financial reward have already influenced researchers to exaggerate positive results and hide risks, just as with antidepressants.[7] And so, at the advent of the so-called 'Shroom Boom',[8] an industry pro-jected to reach \$10.75 billion by 2027,[9] we need to ask the same questions as we did about the decade of the brain: is this the alternative to the old psychiatric drugs it purports to be, or is it the same moot hope in a new guise?

'Woah-man' science

The primary and most visible investor of the John Hopkins centre, Tim Ferriss, stands out among his counterparts. Unlike the other investors, who vest their hopes solely in the potential for one-stop cures, Ferriss thinks that psyche-delics have far broader-reaching potential. In discussing his motivations for his investment in the Johns Hopkins Centre for Psychedelic & Consciousness Research, as well as a previous investment in a similar venture at Imperial College London, he explains that the real excitement, for him, doesn't *just* lie in the 'potential value of psychedelics curing ... psychiatric conditions.'[10] The real possibility is in the fact that, should these conditions prove to be 'close cousins and reflective of certain underlying issues that can be addressed with psychedelics,' this 'changes the entire scope of our understanding of how the mind and psyche functions.'[11]

These are the kind of 'woah, man' statements that I think give flavour to the enthusiasm for psychedelics among researchers, investors and the media. Scepticism regarding the misguided promises drugs have offered in the past is far from the minds of these psychedelic pioneers. To them, these drugs are nothing short of revolutionary.

The very word 'psychedelics' originates from the 1960s countercultural movement. Then, too, the term promised mind-expanding, world-altering perception. Upturning conventional social structures, sexual relations, and hierarchies, counterculture advocated psychedelics as a path to opening people's minds to insanity; not their own, but of the world around them. They were gateways to social change. As Aldous Huxley, the man who popularised psychedelics in the West with his countercultural best-sellers, put it to the psychiatrist Humphry Osmond, who had been working with the hallucinogen mescaline to try to mimic schizophrenia-like states in his research: 'It will give that elixir a bad name if it continues to be associated, in the public mind, with schizophrenia symptoms. People will think they are going mad, when in fact, they are beginning, when they take it, to go sane.'[12] Osmond and Huxley together coined a new term to describe the experience of taking LSD: 'psychedelic', which means 'mind manifesting', and with it, birthed a movement that was about much more than curing mental disease, but about mind-opening potential.

The story of science's embrace of psychedelics, framed in the media as a 'psychedelic renaissance',[13] is couched in a narrative of a return to counterculture. And with it, all the accompanying associations of anti-institutional, anti-hierarchical utopia. The hope of psychedelics contains a hope of manifesting a better world, through the magic of these substances. The emancipatory narrative has been spread far and wide by the media and companies.[14] While scientists were conducting interesting and promising work on psychedelics in the 1940s, most notably with LSD and mescaline, the story goes, the countercultural movement, with its interest in dismantling the rigid boundaries between sanity and madness that psychiatry had guarded, eventually delegitimised psychedelic research within psychiatry. By 1966, the Drug Enforcement Administration had reclassified the drug as a Schedule I substance, with a 'high potential for abuse' and without any 'currently accepted medical use',[15] stymying research. Until the current rush of reanimated interest, that is.

There is much wrong with this narrative, not least, as we'll see, the notion that it was counterculture that derailed psychedelic research in the 1940s, and not the limitations of the research itself. But are these allusions to counterculture, with the psychedelic hope and promise of a better world, now verified (or should we say, co-opted?) by scientific authority? Is this really one for us to hold onto?

Unfortunately, like psychedelics, the emancipatory narrative about counterculture is equally dubious. Even in the 1960s, there was always the question of whose freedom counterculture was manifesting. The movement, for example, posed a contradiction for women. Although it challenged conventional social realities, including sexual relations and the structure of the family, that bound women, and although the movement espoused so-called 'female values' and a 'feminine' way of being, even making them central to a public way of life, quite tellingly the counterculture was not led by women. Rather, it was the beginning of a redefinition, by young men themselves, of the traditional male role.[16] Men were willing to become more 'feminised', but they did not encourage women to assume traditional masculine characteristics and roles. The movement granted women access but made them no more than assistants in a still male-led movement. This is exemplified by the quintessential countercultural literature like Kerouac's *On the Road* that documents the reinvention of manhood for a group of male friends through a journey encompassing sex, drugs, music and roaming around to explore the complexities of freedom; a kind of freedom that depended on a cast of subsidiary female characters as the anchors and security in their supposed rejection of traditional family structures.

Today, too, we should be wary of who the turn to psychedelics will actually benefit. A sense of social exclusivity is already felt in the macho proclamations of high-profile Silicon Valley executives and entrepreneurs, who have publicly shared their fearless personal journeys of 'overcoming' (on expensive trips to remote locations) – the likes of Tim Ferriss, or venture capitalist Ben Horowitz, following in the footsteps of Steve Jobs. In discussions alluding to the world-changing potential of these substances, however, there is little actual talk, in concrete terms, of the social change that would be required to foster better mental health across society. Instead, these psychedelic discussions seem to have displaced any possibility of social change, with another shiny, and highly marketable, misnomer. Despite Ferriss' emphasis that psychedelics are not to be thought of 'just as' cures, this continues to be the salient narrative, and the potential of cures for predefined diseases continues to be at the heart of investors' motivations. There continues to be a lot of discussion between powerful, predominantly White and male investors and scientists, about the exciting potential of this new field and industry, rather than discussions about who gets access and at what cost, or about the social conditions that make talk of 'cures' necessary in the first place, or about the broader sense of wellbeing that might exist outside of this streamlined vision of disease and cure.

Peer through the haze of psychiatry's psychedelic lightshow, and there is still a psychiatric profession drawing on new 'scientific' hopes that attract investment and prestige. There are still investors spreading unrealistic expectations of what these 'fixes' can do, while people's real problems are neglected. And, we will see, there is also a wasted opportunity to learn from psychedelic practices about what and who psychiatry is currently missing.

The narrow view

Let's return to the founding story of psychedelic medicine. The magic mushroom, that emblem of psychedelics and the counterculture, has become a promising compound in the new psychedelic psychiatry. These mushrooms contain the psychoactive compound psilocybin, which has been demonstrated in several studies, combining its use with therapy, to decrease symptoms of depression[17] and anxiety[18] and assist in the treatment of addiction.[19] The story propagated by the media would have us believe that the origins of this treatment in psychiatry lie with the Swiss chemist Albert Hofmann, who in 1958, isolated psilocybin in the laboratory. But as ever, there is another version of history, revealing a less linear, less western and less patriarchal truth.

There is another story, about how the Mazatec native healer María Sabina had introduced her psilocybin mushroom-based practice to author and ethnomycologist R. Gordon Wasson.[20] Wasson studied how Sabina led religious ceremonies and rituals in her native Mexico,[21] then wrote about his experiences with Sabina in what would become a seminal 1957 *Life magazine* article, 'Seeking the Magic Mushroom'. He has become known as the 'father of ethnomycology', referring to his role in the rise of western counterculture's interest in psychedelics.[22] The spores that Wasson identified as *Psilocybe mexicana* went on to be cultivated in Europe, before Hofmann eventually isolated psilocybin in his laboratory – another 'founding father' of western psychedelics, only now in a scientific context. All derived from the practices of Mazatec healing culture that Sabina had shared with Wasson.

In the hands of western medicine, the practices of indigenous[23] people are erased and reduced to biological compounds, which in themselves are said to contain all the magic of restoration and healing. But unearthing these hidden histories of psychedelic medicine reveals the context in which these substances were used. The attempts to reframe psychedelics as a credible science today, displaces the knowledge and practices of the traditions they came from, drawing on and reinforcing the widespread western cultural belief that scientific knowledge is superior, along with the western cultures and people at its centre. Take Ferriss, who continues to laud the mind-expanding opportunities of psychedelics, while distancing himself from its source, in an attempt to prop up the new, 'proper', scientific foundation of his business ventures. He describes, for example, how he was inspired by the Buddhist psychologist Tara Brach, and refers to her 'outstanding book called *Radical Acceptance*', but, Ferriss makes sure to mention that the book 'was recommended to me by a neuroscience PhD who is as anti-woo-woo as possible.'[24] Brach is American, and considered a western teacher of Buddhism; even this, it seems, was considered too close to the source.

This isn't just an ethical point about the cultural appropriation through which western medicine has drawn on the knowledge of other cultures for capital gain (while barring these communities from the practices they had invented by legalising commodified variants). This is also about the efficacy of these purported miracle cures when transplanted without their cultural context. Sabina's use of psilocybin was part of a practice of chanting through the night. She was able to effectively heal because people participated in this ritual, which in their cultural context, had meaning. The ritual and context are an important dimension, an enabling dimension, in fact, of the mushrooms' healing effect. As we'll soon see, a person's commitment to change, expressed through ritual, is probably the most powerful component of any psychedelic 'recovery'. But all of this was lost in the western translation of laboratory-synthesised psilocybin that entered western markets.

Without a suitable social context, synthesised replicas won't work.

For all the claims of investors about the miraculous properties of their isolated psychedelic substances today, their medical benefits have only ever been proven *in combination with* therapy. The context of the experience, these studies show, is paramount. Recreational drug users know this, too: the importance of 'set', or a person's mindset as they enter a psychedelic experience, ideally relaxed and free of fear, as well as 'setting', which should be an environment that feels comfortable and safe. When these are off, you're likely to have a bad trip. It makes sense that the converse would also be true.

Studies on the efficacy of psychedelic treatment emphasise the importance of set and setting, in addition to a comfortable therapeutic clinician-patient relationship to facilitating healing experiences and realising positive outcomes.[25] There is a wealth of history that teaches us more than the latest boon in psychiatric articles about the necessary conditions for psychedelic healing. This perspective is precluded, however, in a scientific industry interested in patentable drugs with a conventionally scientific, biological mechanism; drugs that 'work' generically, regardless of their context, so that they can be sold as one-size-fits-all products.

In fact, terms like 'set' and 'setting' appearing in the psychiatric literature point to the limits of the biomedical model in explaining the role of psychedelics in healing. The terms are deployed to describe 'extra-pharmacological' variables; effects that cannot be reduced to chemical action, that cannot be framed as part of the intellectual property, the drug, the chemical compound, that companies are selling. These terms are researchers' way of trying to control the psychedelic narrative. It is in their best interest, of course, to find a language capable of reducing the highly context-dependent effects of psychedelics to a marketable product, to a formula that promises results, thus attracting the funding of those enthusiastic investors.

Pharmaceutical start-ups flooding the psychedelic space are trying hard to make psychedelics conform to the pharmaceutical formula of biological disease with chemical cure. Researchers continue to create new compounds which are not psychoactive, but similar to psychedelic compounds, which they can then patent, and whose effects they can purport to know precisely, predict and control – unlike the recreational drugs used outside the medical context. This lands us in that same bizarre situation that we have seen across the pharmaceutical industry, in which drug manufacturers with no clinical experience, detached from the actual context in which these drugs are used, make grand claims about the efficacy and safety of their products. By providing supposedly tightly controlled, legitimate alternatives, appropriating terms like 'set' and 'setting' to mop up the effects they cannot control or explain, they claim these ancient substances, making them legal and available for a small group of people at hefty prices. This is a tense tightrope act. You only have to look at the increasingly absurd array of non-biological components these companies are trying to draw into their patents – patents on basic elements of the psychedelic experience, or patents covering dozens of possible conditions that might be treatable[26] – to see how they are struggling to maintain their monopoly on healing the mind. And in doing so, we are all missing an opportunity to widen our view of the healing process, and understand the role that the right environmental conditions and supportive care can bring.

Psychedelic visions

The highly individualised nature of effective psychedelic therapy is where it offers not just a vision of psychiatry infused with a new chemical, but a new way of doing psychiatry altogether. Choice, here, is determinant of how effective a ritual will be; a person's commitment to a particular ritual, and a context for the ritual they have chosen and given form to. If that is the case, the role of the psychiatrist, whether they are working with psychedelics or antidepressants, should be less about administering treatment, and more about facilitating a context in which a person can make sense of their life experiences. Combined with what we now know about the social determinants of mental distress, we could extend this role for psychiatrists beyond administering drugs, to one of coordinating support that addresses the various, proven, causes of mental suffering: to help people with financial difficulties, housing, finding social support groups, or accessing culturally embedded care that is consistent with how they understand their mental suffering. Psychiatrists could help people piece together a combination of support, from drugs to social groups to safety plans, that make sense to them. To do this, psychiatrists will have to take up their place in a system that connects them to other, equally valuable, mental health offerings. They will need to prioritise building relationships with other services, and also, crucially, with the people they are trying to help, above asserting their medical expertise.

Psychiatrists may even enjoy this way of working more. I spoke with the founders and current organisers of Intentional Peer Support (IPS), an organisation that advocates for equal, reciprocal relationships as an alternative to the hierarchical doctor-patient dynamic. The team told me about the impact their work had had on medical staff in hospitals, and in many cases, they noticed drastic shifts in how clinicians saw their role. This extended beyond simply understanding more intimately the harm that coercion causes patients. Clinicians had a newfound willingness and understanding of how important connection is with people who are suffering. Initially focused on making a diagnosis and prescribing medication, by the end of the training, people were, according to Lisa Archibald, the UK-based co-director at IPS, 'actually taking time to see the person and to be interested in their experience.' With this, Archibald said, came an appreciation of the views and inputs of people using the services. But the training also helped clinicians imagine themselves with a new responsibility; not just as experts, but also as people with their own experience. Their personal lives were no longer something to hide as they performed the role of sane expert in relation to the insane patient. Their experience with life's difficulties became an important asset, a qualification for the job, now that they understood that job to be centrally about building relationships.

Archibald told me how many clinicians made career changes after their training, deciding to become peer workers because they found the work so meaningful. These 'converts' talked about how differently they viewed the people they worked with in their new role. While working on acute wards as clinicians, they repeatedly said, they only saw people at their worst. They didn't see people in between admissions, when they were coping or doing well, and this gave them a distorted view of people as always struggling, as completely suffering. This is another consequence of a system based on diagnosis and cure. People are defined and treated in a narrow capacity that reduces them to patients, and erases everything else they are. And this leads to assumptions and limited estimations of a person's potential. Any system that operates in the shadow of a totalising diagnosis, will miss important opportunities to relate to the parts of a person that are well, and their capacity for survival as well as positive change.

It is no wonder that some clinicians eventually choose to work in a peer support capacity, where they get to build longer-term relationships that give them a fuller sense of a person's ebbs and flows, rather than a problem to be diagnosed. This seems like more fulfilling work. In any case, a perspective that prioritises relationships with patients as people, will begin to shift the medical world's understanding of their role in what needs to be a multi-faceted system of care.

A different healing story

For all their legal reaching and neologisms, psychedelics refuse to be contained. People continue to seek out psychedelic experiences beyond the medical context – indeed, they seek them out precisely because the experience takes them out of the medical context.

This comes with risks. But what the medical model of drugs with its supposedly predictable outcomes, administered in tightly controlled clinical settings, fails to acknowledge, is that a certain degree of unpredictability can actually be key to the process of healing. Cultural historian and author Mike Jay, who has written extensively on psychedelics, told me that he had seen some miraculous cases of psychedelic healing in contexts that a doctor would never have put a patient into. 'But that's also a part of it,' he said. Indigenous rituals involving psychedelics are premised on that same notion of a journey, of disruptive process that also challenges the limits of your own self-perception, and of your life's possibilities. This is how Jay explains the rise of ayahuasca tourism to the Amazon – people are seeking solutions specifically outside the clinical paradigm because they offer what he calls 'a different kind of recovery narrative'. The journey provides an intentional ritual that is meaningful to the individual, a story that allows them to make a commitment to change, allows them to integrate that change into their identity by claiming it as part of their life story. That decision is empowering and is as important as the actual substance taken.

Though they may be transformative, these experiences, once again, likely don't reach those who need them most. The recovery narratives aided by psychedelic retreats are, of course, privy to marketisation, just like bankrolled pharmaceuticals. As part of a rising wellness industry, the customer base for psychedelic retreats is the affluent 'experience-seeking consumer'; these experiences are inaccessible to most people, and especially those who are most in need of psychiatric care.

Nonetheless, the psychedelic experience can show us a new role for the drugs and people involved in medical treatment for mental health problems. People who suffer from extreme mental states like deep depression or psychosis, have been exposed to the uncertainty of life. Their confidence in the bounds of reality, or their ability to control their own reality, has been profoundly shaken. A drug, administered by an expert usurping control over their lives, might actually reinforce that sense of powerlessness. An experience someone chooses, on the other hand, might restore this sense of trust in their own ability to survive. This requires approaches that restore a sense of connectedness, empowerment, identity, meaning, hope and optimism *in the face of uncertainty*; a kind of confidence rooted in a base belief that we will handle whatever comes.[27] A psychedelic experience can give people an opportunity to challenge the limits of their own self-estimation, growing a sense of confidence, rooted in a strong connection with themselves and the world around them, that they can survive. This effect does not just flow from a chemical into a bloodstream; it requires immersion in a process of experiencing and ongoing reflection, as people find ways to integrate the *experience* of taking the drug into their lives – claiming the ritual as part of their life stories, so that it becomes a vehicle for meaningful change. This also explains the long-lasting positive effects psilocybin can have on personality traits such as openness to experience and emotional stability.[28] In the studies on

psilocybin so far, subjects often report that their experience taking the drug is challenging, but that the effects are
long-lasting, meaningful and life-changing.[29] The chemical compound may facilitate this experience, but it is a
tool in a process that is centrally about human agency in
the face of life's unknown.

Research on mental health therapies more generally
confirms the importance of commitment and agency to
healing, showing that a meaningful ritual is important
across the board when recovering from mental distress.
What this ritual is makes fairly little difference to recovery
rates: no matter what kind of therapy, spiritual practice
or prescribed drug-taking ritual people choose, if they are
committed to it and believe in it, the results are comparable.[30] In this context, the role of psychedelics is comparable
to that of hypnotherapy: both are about making talking
therapy more immersive, and so more effective, but neither
can be passively administered to manifest healing. It isn't
difficult to imagine how emerging triumphant from a
turbulent shamanic ritual is more transformative than: 'I
went to the doctor and was given a new prescription.' This
model for recovery does not gel with the controlled, clinical western context for a 'cure', but it might be much more
effective for some.

It makes sense, of course, that those at the forefront of
psychedelic entrepreneurship want to project a scientific
certainty – psychedelics is a young field in need of funding
to build a research base that is considered medically legitimate. Scientific certainty that presents itself as a safe bet,
as we saw earlier, attracts funding. One review, published
in August 2022, that studied how adverse events in psychedelics research have been flagged, found that they have
been inconsistently and, likely, underreported.[31] Many

trials reported no adverse effects whatsoever – an unlikely reality, and one that seeks to control a scientific narrative based on irrefutable facts and promises. This kind of objectivity, long the aim of psychiatric science, misconstrues the process.

Psychedelics can be incredibly healing, as many experiences, (including the many that go unreported in the annals of psychedelic medicine) will attest, but this is not a generic prescription. In fact, studies have shown that the psychedelic 'treatment' *has to be* personalised to have any impact at all. Psychiatry will have to accept the limitations of its prescriptive power if it is to make any real contributions to psychedelic healing. It will have to allow its narrative to be changed by psychedelics; to embrace a new role, not as an arbiter of pills, but as a guide in personalised and person-led care. Psychiatrists could begin to imagine their role as one of facilitating choice, to empower an individual to heal, rather than prescribing them a generic cure. Perhaps there is a version of a mental healthcare system, for example, in which rather than prescribing a drug or treatment, psychiatrists present people with detailed information on medical and non-medical therapies and allow them to choose the ritual that is most meaningful to them. Indeed, this approach to delivery is being trialled in the Netherlands at the time of writing.[32] The true revolutionary power of psychedelics doesn't lie in the hope of a cure as psychiatry has long defined it, but in how it might open up new ways of doing psychiatry itself.

Psychedelic power

Psychedelics has entered mainstream psychiatry. This is not a time for blind faith. This is an opportunity to redefine the relationships that shape the field: between doctors and patients, between classes, between ethnicities, and between different parts of the world. This is about looking beyond a miracle cure, marketed as a generic cure for anyone (with the money to pay for it), and instead focusing on placing more importance on the context in which these are used. But the association between psychedelics and counterculture can also help draw attention to psychiatry's wider context: the social disparity that determines who gets to benefit from the kinds of environments that could make drug use beneficial.

The case of psychedelics shows us that the lines between legal and illegal drugs is political. Nothing has changed about psychedelics themselves in the years since counterculture, only the people taking them; once marginalised 'hippies', now powerful billionaires. And that should remind us to look to the broader social context in which psychedelics are used, to understand who benefits from them today.

A 1994 interview with Nixon's domestic policy advisor, John Ehrlichman, that resurfaced in a 2016 *Harper's Magazine* article,[33] and most recently in Michael Pollan's 2021 book *This is Your Mind on Plants*,[34] reminded us of the political power vested in these divides. In the interview, Ehrlichman explained the motivations driving America's drug war:

The Nixon campaign in 1968, and the Nixon White House after that, had two enemies: the antiwar left and black people ... We knew we couldn't make it illegal to be either against the war or black, but by getting the public to associate hippies with marijuana and blacks with heroine, and then criminalising both heavily, we could disrupt those communities. We could arrest their leaders, raid their homes, break up their meetings, and vilify them night after night on the evening news. Did we know we were lying about the drugs? Of course we did.[35]

However definitive Ehrlichman's judgement of Nixon's policy was, the interview highlighted the power that was being asserted in the state response to the American drug problem in the US. Heroin use had become more widespread among young Black men in the 1950s, very much driven by poverty and discrimination. Rather than offering social support, the government opted for a primarily legal and punitive response, and this has only intensified since. In the United States, the opioid epidemic – more prevalent among White Americans – was declared a 'national public health emergency'[36] by Trump and led to tolerant incarceration-avoidant programmes for White opioid users, while such an approach has not been considered for drugs more common in Black communities.[37] There were no such efforts to resolve the crack epidemic of the 1980s, for example, which mostly impacted poor African Americans; instead, African American crack users were imprisoned at astonishing rates.[38] Today, people of colour and people with low economic status in countries across the world continue to be disproportionately incarcerated for possession of drugs.[39] [40] African Americans in particular continue to be more likely to be arrested, receive harsher punishment, and face longer sentences than whites, although they use drugs at roughly the same rate.[41]

The very real sense of fear that this criminalisation fosters in the populations it targets is likely difficult for members of these communities to reconcile with the sense of enthusiasm espoused by psychedelic researchers. Add to this a history of medical racism that has exploited and abused Black people and other people of colour,[42] [43] and it is understandable that they may not feel inclined to participate in psychedelic clinical trials or submit to treatment.[44] This has resulted in a dearth of studies on ways in which psychedelics can be used to target the specificities of the traumas experienced by these groups of people.[45] In a recent review of 17 international psychedelic studies conducted from 2000 to 2017, 82.5 per cent of participants were White. Overall, rates of recruitment of people of colour in psychedelic medicine are very low.[46] Knowing, in addition to this, the mental health consequences of longstanding discrimination, how revolutionary can a psychedelic science be for mental health when it excludes the groups of people most affected by the social causes of mental distress?

The political context of drug criminalisation reminds us that new drugs do not offer real hope for social change when they exist in the same racist, sexist and classist systems as the old drugs. They just offer more of the same. While its advocates present psychedelics as a revolution in mental healthcare, in actual practice, scientific psychedelics as it stands – as an expensive, cutting-edge treatment – offers a therapeutic alternative (among many other existing alternatives) for a small group of people who already have private healthcare insurance. Even as the drivers of the psychedelic renaissance discuss new possible therapeutic paradigms and the questions of access,[47] it remains clear who the arbiters of power in the field are. You only need to look at the constitution of the field to see clearly how this scientific hierarchy of knowledge facilitates the exclusion of voices and reinforces White male domination. The editorial board of the new *Journal of Psychedelic Studies*, published by Wolters Kluwer, is 78 per cent male and also overwhelmingly White.[48] Of all the board members and directors and scientific advisors of the top funding agencies for all psychedelic research internationally, 90 per cent are White men, even though women, non-binary and trans people make up more than half of the clinicians, research staff, volunteers and visionaries guiding these institutions. Most psychedelic research groups, conferences and community events are headlined and led by men, even though social activists, attendees and organisers are mainly women.[49]

Even if treatment was accessible more broadly, for large groups of the population, their disenfranchisement in the medical system is likely to make them sceptical of another treatment delivered in the same way. And with good reason. It will be difficult for them to vest hope in a system that doesn't take seriously the real problems of a historic neglect and mistreatment at the hands of psychiatrists, or the very real problems of poverty, violence and discrimination, none of which will be 'cured' by a new drug that targets the mind, rather than social disparity, no matter how psychedelic the experience.

The 'new science' of psychedelics offers exciting potential to challenge the way psychiatry is done, to shift the focus from finding chemical solutions to new forms of individualised support and structural change in how care is delivered. At the same time, psychedelics are at risk of being (and, to some extent, already have been) drawn into an existing profit-driven system that benefits the rich, White and male. If, however, we follow the insights offered by those psychedelic experiences people identify as useful, we can find in it the vision of mental healthcare based on equal, empowering, culturally attuned and person-centric support. Getting there will require new forms of collaboration, listening and repair. Western psychedelic medicine will need to take responsibility for the systemic inequities it perpetuates through exclusion and the power relationships it creates in the consultation room and beyond. It will have to acknowledge the limitations of current treatment protocols for ethnic minority populations, and also its role in cultural appropriation as it continues to patent practices that exclude the populations that created them.[50] It will have to value, and include, the knowledge of groups of people and areas of study that fall outside of neuroscience. And it will have to involve the people currently placed on the passive side of the relationship between psychiatrist and patient, in shaping care that works for them. This is a far cry from the vision of miracle cures promised by a new psychedelic research centre; it's a vision that's complex, varied, highly individual and ever-changing. But there is also a simplicity in its goal to empower individual people to live their lives. This system would be anchored in a principle of minimising power disparities between those offering and those seeking support.

8

Neurodiversity as a Model for Care

We've now explored in detail the perils of biological explanations of mental distress, in particular through the lens of neuroscience, as well as the limits of diagnosis. Repeatedly, we've raised the question of what a language that more accurately reflects the experience and (social) causes of mental distress might look like, a language that still communicates a person's needs and can be used to access and design support.

While some critics argue for a less medical vocabulary for mental health, others argue that we simply need to destigmatise the current one. Neurodivergence has emerged as a term to describe a difference in how some people's brains process information. This very much echoes, then, the dominant medical explanations of mental experiences being largely brain-related. Diagnoses like autism, attention deficit disorder (ADHD), dyslexia and dyspraxia are typically included in the bracket of neurodivergence. Many who identify as neurodiverse argue that these labels do not connote a deficit in the person; while they recognise the real difficulties of living in a world that doesn't cater for difference in mental processing, they argue that it is this world, not neurodiverse individuals, that need correcting. By normalising difference, and proudly wearing these labels, this approach challenges societal ideas about psychiatric diagnosis as a whole. Others believe that adopting this language only reinforces the legitimacy of a medically dominant language that stigmatises and misrepresents the diversity of experience across the population, and falls short in meeting their needs.

There are no straightforward answers, but there is definitely a lot to learn from the history of conditions like autism, where those diagnosed have found an increasingly audible voice. Autism has been at the centre of the discussions about neurodivergence, which are very much about the aims, interests and power vested in psychiatric research and treatment. Activism around autism has challenged many of the assumptions that, as we've seen, have implicitly driven diagnosis and treatment in so many areas of research. Assumptions around equating 'normality' with health, the idea that medical cures are preferable to social ones, and, indeed, whether cures are needed at all. Autism activists have also raised questions about whose voices should drive priorities in research – from parent advocates to autistic people themselves (who have, in turn, sometimes been in conflict). Activists have critiqued autism research, pointing to the exclusion of women from studies, an over-emphasis on the deficits of autistic people, and generally having aims that don't reflect the needs and priorities of people living with autism. These discussions challenge the power structures that have governed psychiatry for so long, drawing attention to the experiential knowledge, and obvious support psychiatry might be missing. Crucially, they also show how many solutions arise, easily, when we involve people affected in designing research and care.

Autistic women

Since the release of *Rain Man* in 1989, the cultural understanding of autism has featured a cast of quirky and obsessive but usually highly functioning individuals, often with exceptional talents. Film characters have been very influential in shaping public understandings of autism; the idea that autism is accompanied by exceptional 'savant' abilities in a particular area, like extraordinary memory, is still a widespread belief.[1] But these film characters aren't representative of the reality of autism in all its variations. They do not show audiences the joys, challenges and range of experiences of autistic people, and fail to ask what it would mean not just to accept but learn from and respond to their experiences. Instead, all are tinged with 'redeeming' qualities that make them more relatable to mainstream audiences. The implication here is that the usual 'able-bodied' person is a norm to aspire to. And perhaps it is that vie for cultural acceptance that explains another common denominator connecting the cast of 'autistic' characters populating our cultural consciousness. They are, of course, all men.

Not much is known, historically, about autistic women – although that is now thankfully changing.[2] This is because it isn't just in the media where autistic women have been strangely absent; in psychiatry, too, researchers refer to these women as 'research orphans'. Autism is diagnosed about 4 times as often in men as it is in women. Many autistic women are initially misdiagnosed with something else. Anything from anxiety disorders, depression and mood disorders, borderline personality disorder, to eating disorders.[3]

It is not difficult to see how the traits associated with autism spectrum disorder (ASD), as it is known today, do not jive with culturally sanctioned femininity. The criteria in the DSM-5, released in 2013, and updated in 2022, for diagnosing ASD include three key areas of difficulty in social communication and social interactions. To be diagnosed with ASD, an individual must experience difficulties in 'social emotional reciprocity', which includes, for example, trouble with approaching someone for an interaction, back and forth conversation, sharing interests with others, and expressing or understanding emotions. They must also have difficulties in using and understanding nonverbal communication, including eye contact, body language, facial expressions or gestures. They must struggle in developing and maintaining relationships with other people, including a lack of apparent interest in others, difficulties responding to different social contexts, and difficulties in sharing imaginative play with others. In addition, individuals must demonstrate another two of four restricted and repetitive behaviours, interests or activities, including things like a strict adherence to routines, very particular and extreme interests or an unusual interest in certain sensory aspects of the environment, like specific sounds or textures.[4]

Much of this behaviour, for women, transgresses gender lines. Women are supposed to be sociable and group-oriented, rather than individualistic and obsessive; the latter is the realm of male lone-wolf geniuses. Women are meant to be caring, and maintain social harmony, and definitely not disrupt it. They are meant to be more about emotions and less about ideas and interests. It is easy to see how, culturally, it is difficult to reconcile 'femininity' with autism. And psychiatry doesn't hover objectively above those cultural ideas, as we've seen throughout this book; gender stereotypes shape ideas about normality that guide the questions researchers ask, the treatment psychiatrists offer, and, also, who gets treatment at all.

So, it is hopeful that the cultural face of autism is changing, showing us how the social forces shaping men and women affect them mentally in particular ways.

The gender gap in diagnosing autism has indisputably risen to the fore in recent years. A slew of reporting has spurred this on, largely spotlighting celebrity and personal testimonials that state and try to explain gender differences in presentation and diagnosis for women, as opposed to men. In 2021 English TV presenter Melanie Sykes spoke about the relief of receiving a diagnosis at fifty-one. Her story was presented as part of a trend of women increasingly being diagnosed with autism spectrum disorder in adulthood.[5] For Sykes, the diagnosis was 'life-changing' and helped her make sense of the previously inexplicable struggles she had faced. This news was optimistic in tone, attributing the rising diagnostic rates to a growing awareness that autism is not, as was previously believed, a male disease. The differences in the way that autism presents in women is increasingly much better understood,[6] and journalists point to the shifting male-to-female ratio of autism diagnosis as evidence of progress. In 1998, 18 per cent of new diagnoses in England were women, in 2018, it was 23 per cent.[7] In the US, too, newspapers reported a similar increase in diagnoses. In 2012, boys were 4.7 times as likely as girls to be diagnosed with autism, by 2018, they were only 4.2 times as likely, and in 2023, this had dropped to 3.8.[8]

Much of the hope in the media comes from more equal gender representation in clinical samples of neuroscience and genetics studies. Until recently, women weren't included, for example, in the neuro-imaging studies that provided instructive insights into the brains of autistic men. Diagnostic criteria were skewed towards identifying autism in men because, until recently, most scientific studies recruited only boys and men. It was a self-sustaining logic, where autism was believed to be more common in boys than in girls, and so scientists only studied boys. Things are changing now, journalists relay, because more money had become available for cutting-edge science on gender differences in autism.[9]

We now know, of course, that many of the supposedly cutting-edge findings in psychiatry remain inconclusive for men and women alike. The studies on gender differences in autism, too, have been overall inconclusive, and with limited utility in guiding diagnosis. In early studies, for example, scientists hopefully pursued genetic explanations that would distil the differences in the prevalence of autism to a difference in genes. A boy might carry a mutation in his DNA on his single X chromosome that leads to autism, whereas a girl who inherits the same mutation would be unaffected because she has a second X chromosome to compensate. Scientists never found an X-factor. The search for genetic factors continues, with new theories emerging that propose that women's DNA has a protective effect against mutations causing autism. A 2012 paper that laid out this 'female protective effect' in autism marked a turning point in the field, and drew much scientific attention to gender differences in autism.[10] A group of scientists in the same year were awarded a five-year, $13 million grant to probe the differences between autistic girls and boys,[11] investigating the differences in behaviour, genetics, brain structure and function. As ever, the hope that biology would illuminate the mental experience shone luminescent. But with all this money going into understanding the biology of autism, results remain underwhelming, to the point where prominent researchers are speaking out about the lack of applicable findings in autism research.[12]

The most helpful understanding about gender differences, it turns out, has not come from neuroscience, but from studies that are more directly applicable to clinicians trying to make a diagnosis. These tend to be studies on the lived experience of autistic people, rather than their genes or brains.

Social differences

Many of the differences between autistic boys and girls align uncannily with the differences between boys and girls *in general*. Autistic girls are, for example, chattier, less disruptive, and less interested in vehicles than boys are. This is also typically true of girls and boys more broadly, and so it becomes difficult to separate gender differences in autism from gender differences in general.[13] Considering the gendered pressures we have named throughout this book, it isn't really uncanny resemblance, so much as common sense reasoning, that autistic people are subject to the same socialisation and social pressures as anyone else. These findings simply remind us that we cannot understand mental variation in a scientific vacuum, however advanced the tools might be, and need to look, once again, to the social world to understand the meaning of people's experiences.

Studies are now starting to document the role of gender-related pressures in the social lives of autistic people. These studies echo the findings that gender differences in diagnosis are inflated; that women have autism much more than was previously recognised. But the explanations offered for these missed diagnoses is based less on the state of the science, than clinicians' lack of knowledge about the social lives of girls and women. Girls are socialised in a way that teaches them to mask their symptoms in ways that boys do not: to make eye contact when speaking, for example, to laugh and make others feel at ease. Girls in general are encouraged to display this kind of conciliatory behaviour, and so it isn't entirely surprising that autistic girls notice these patterns and learn to copy the girls and women around them.[14]

Yet camouflage only goes so far. Often, it carries autistic girls up to the point of adolescence. As they enter their teens, autistic girls struggle to keep up with the elaborate rules of social relationships. Many girls learn to imitate their peers, copying their mannerisms to blend in, at great cost to their inner selves. The intricacies of teenage girls' social codes often leave autistic girls confused, exhausted and isolated. This is in contrast to adolescent autistic boys who tend to socialise in loosely organised groups centred around activities. This makes it easier for a boy with different social abilities to join in. Among teenage girls, socialisation revolves around a different form of communication. Bonds are consolidated by discussing relationships among the group, for example, or talking about emotions.[15] These social pressures may not be felt in the same way by all autistic girls – for example, we cannot assume that they will feel the same for those who are completely non-verbal. But for many autistic girls, there are particular complexities that reflect how they are gendered. They are likely to be aware that they are being excluded but may not understand why. This might lead to a sense of inadequacy and personal failure, which, combined with isolation, is a toxic cocktail for our state of mind. This is, of course, in addition to (or is just another version of) the sense of inadequacy and personal failure many teenage girls already experience as a result of the self-policing and comparisons they are socialised into.

But for many autistic women, the issues they face have everything to do with their gender. That is, not their biological sex, but the social repercussions of their gender nonconformity in our social world. There are particular challenges most autistic women will face, and we have to draw light to these in research and society to develop care that responds to these women's needs. Autistic women face the same social world as most women, and will struggle, differently, but struggle all the same. How can we help autistic women deal with puberty and menstruation? To navigate the codes of female friendships? To talk about romance and sexuality? How can we help them stay safe in a world that presents a higher risk for interpersonal violence to women and genderqueer people?

Even after a girl gets the right diagnosis, she is likely to receive the same support boys do; a one-size-fits-all policy, except that that one size was designed specifically with men in mind. Behavioural therapy is a go-to, just as with the personality disorders like BPD, and the logic behind this is the same. The therapy teaches autistic people methods of assimilation – to make eye contact or turn to the person they are speaking to. This only goes so far, for anyone, given that a person's developmental and emotional needs cannot be met simply by learning to 'fit in' and mask their experience. Yet it is true that being a woman demands, at the very least, a different skillset to form connection and friendship, and to feel safe and empowered in the world. Scientists and service providers rarely acknowledge the additional challenges being an autistic woman brings, and so the issues for autistic women proliferate. Starting in childhood, depression, anxiety and eating disorders are more common for autistic girls and women than autistic boys and men.[16] But these other symptoms might also help to explain how other conditions are often diagnosed first for girls; they might distract doctors from the autistic traits. At the same time, some of these diagnoses contrast less starkly with notions of femininity, or at best, frame these behaviours as the social transgressions they are deemed to be, such as anxiety, depression or borderline personality disorder.

An interview with Caroline Logan, a consultant forensic clinical psychologist in the UK's National Health Service gave me insight into the most extreme consequences of misdiagnosis of autism. She told me how autistic people are not infrequently misdiagnosed with psychopathy, given that empathic deficit is a core symptom of both disorders. In autism spectrum disorders there is sometimes antisocial behaviour which could be caused partly by incorrect evaluation of social situations, or perhaps a combination of frustration and anger resulting from difficulties in social contexts. In psychopathy, of course, the antisocial behaviour often involves insensitive manipulation and exploitation of another person. Given the difficulty of diagnosing women with psychopathy, this is incredibly murky territory, and we have to wonder, in any case, how often a woman's nonconforming experience is punished, rather than understood. The costs of misdiagnosis will be disastrous in whichever direction it occurs, both for the woman herself, who might risk, for example, punitive treatment, sectioning, or even incarceration if her social confusion leads to violence, rather than help in understanding herself and those around her.[17]

A caveat here, is that the social explanations of the underdiagnosis of autism in women risk repeating the same assumptions and mistakes in medical approaches that group and pathologise nonconformity to a perceived 'norm'. Again, we cannot generalise about the experience of autistic women as if their experience is generic, especially considering the whole spectrum of experiences that may, for example, also involve seizures, repetitive behaviours, being non-verbal and other cognitive processing differences. We cannot assume a norm, just as we cannot generalise about the experience of women, in general ignoring their intersectionality, or individual uniqueness. Every autistic person will have a different experience, and not all of them will regard that experience as problematic. We will discuss later how self-advocacy in autism has begun to reframe autism as a unique and equally legitimate human experience, in contrast to a medical, deficit-based view that regards autism as a disorder to be fixed. While in a world designed for neurotypical people, autistic people may require special support, this should not imply that they are ill or deficient. While autistic women are likely to face some similar societal barriers as autistic men, it is essential that we respond to women's needs as they see them, rather than 'curing' them by bringing them in line with ideas of normal gender-typical behaviour. With the former perspective, studies on gender-specific presentations of autism can provide a useful tool; with the latter, they become a reinvented mechanism of oppression.

The biological hope returns

The growing public awareness and media surrounding autistic celebrities and women could mean that more autistic women receive a diagnosis that might help them make sense of the difficulties they face in navigating a world built both for men and for people without autism. Many have stated the clarifying and affirming consequence of their diagnosis. Yet this is not always a given. Much of the research foregrounded in current articles is the brain studies and genetic insights that promise (but have yet to) explain the differences between the presentation between autism in men and women. As interesting as this research may be, given the palpable difficulties autistic women face in the social world, it is this latter kind of research that needs to be prioritised. What we see in the current media attention to autistic women, is an all-too-easy return to the biological hope narrative. The biological hope that, as it did for schizophrenia and depression, promises to cure our minds' ailments with its high-tech innovation.

As ever, that hope is over-stated – we are not as far as media reports make out – and, in addition to that, it obfuscates an important, alternative, source of hope. The hopeful insight is not necessarily that women are different from men when it comes to autism, but the recognition that social worlds impact our mental wellbeing. Perhaps this is the cutting-edge insight we need to follow and invest our research funds into. Because this is where we can make a big difference to people's wellbeing – men, women, or anyone. The hopeful insight and turning point, for a different form of care, is that one-stop solutions are inadequate and not in the best interest of people in general. And, once again, a crucial point is entirely missing: autistic people might not need curing at all.

Just as with other medical conditions, we seem to have a difficult time in straying from the idea of a biological 'cure' for autism. Even the social insights into the lived experience of autistic women are repeatedly presented as biological breakthroughs, couched in biological findings to legitimise them, without much indication of how they will shape actual treatment. The 'camouflaging' women do in social situations, for example, is a behavioural observation long made by clinicians, with neuroscience not really adding too much to the picture. Yet no article is complete without reference to the brain-based differences between men and women.[18] One article that interestingly does acknowledge that neuroscientific findings haven't revealed anything clinically significant[19] cites an interview with Kevin Pelphrey, a professor at the Yale Child Study Center. Pelphrey discusses a multisite project he is leading that promises to make headway into learning how autistic girls are different from boys – both by recording their behaviour and by scanning their brains. The study investigates that oft-cited observation in autistic people, that they are 'uninterested in' or at least 'disengaged from' social interactions. This seems like an unscientific premise, as it assumes a level of disinterest that may simply reveal a way of relating that is *different* but no less interested, but in any case, Pelphrey's brain-imaging evidence revealed that what is implied to be a social deficiency is only true for autistic boys. 'The most surprising thing – it might not be surprising to the clinicians out there, but to the scientists – is that we're seeing strong social-brain activation or function in autistic girls, which is, strictly speaking, counter to everything we've reported ourselves and other groups have reported,' Pelphrey says. 'Their social brains seem to be intact.' Pelphrey's studies revealed that autistic girls are similar to neurotypical boys in how they process social information. One unpublished observation cited in the news article is that, for autistic girls, the social brain

– the interconnected brain regions that manage activities like face processing, emotional processing and tracking people's attention – seems to communicate with the prefrontal cortex, a brain region that normally engages in reason and planning, and is known to burn through energy. It may be that autistic women keep their social brain engaged, but mediate it through the prefrontal cortex – in a sense, intellectualising social interactions that would be intuitive for other women. Essentially, Pelphrey's findings reflect the same 'camouflaging' behaviour observed by clinicians (and no doubt autistic women themselves, as they feel the exhausting effects of socialising) for a long time. The journalist, too, notes that, 'Pelphrey is right that this finding isn't entirely a surprise to clinicians,' that those who regularly see autistic women have picked up on their remarkable ability to learn the rules enough to camouflage their symptoms. Clinicians have had to learn to be creative when diagnosing women on the autism spectrum, rather than simply looking for, say, repetitive behaviour, as they might with men, and relying also on self-reports telling them how stressful it is for women to maintain appearances. Their behavioural adaptations might be so good that these are not a reliable indicator for a diagnosis. All in all, these new brain studies are simply rehashing old insights, and the explanations are far from conclusive; the adaptations girls show could just as well be social mimicry as cognitive compensation.

Of course, it is normal scientific practice to return to questions and to investigate them from different perspectives. But when many women are suffering from the toll of social adaptation, have long been neglected and urgently need support, perhaps a more immediate approach is advisable based on the verified observations that are already available. Currently, the medical paradigm dominated by references to neuroscience leads to the implication that women need to be medically diagnosed; that this is the marker of who needs help. But isn't the current diagnostic method developed by clinicians that includes self-reported stress levels, sufficient? There seems to be an obsession in the current research with improving diagnostic measures; as many scientists put it, 'getting behind the mask' of women who are good at masking their behaviour.[20] With all the enthusiasm for greater visibility of autistic women, is this heightened visibility actually translating into better support? As with all the conditions currently treated with psychotropic drugs, or psychedelics, we need ask whether that visibility is translating into better support, or merely lining the pockets of financial backers and drug companies.

Whose cure?

With the diagnostic tools designed to 'explain' differences between autistic boys and girls, the implication remains that autism is a disorder that needs to be cured. 'Treatment' geared towards 'managing' autism is a flimsy alternative to designing a world that accommodates the needs of neurodiverse people. As with every other diagnosis we have seen, a medical response targets individuals, and entirely sidesteps the possibility of facilitating people's unique experiences rather than targeting 'symptoms' to bring them in line with a perceived normal of a neurotypical world.

But let's ask ourselves: who finds this deviation from the norm problematic? Is it autistic people themselves, or is it instead the people around them? Much of the 'support' currently available for autistic people comes in the form of treatment based on the premise that their abnormal behaviour needs to be brought in line with the norm. While, of course, learning certain social skills might help an autistic person integrate in the social environment they are in, and alleviate some of the social isolation that may be causing them distress, it is unlikely to satisfy their needs and particular interests, because it doesn't support them in the particular way of relating to others and the world around them that is meaningful to them. It is unlikely, too, to register the joy their divergent way of relating to others and the world might bring. Who does this 'cure' really serve? And does the medical model of autism simply conflate cure with conformity?

The true hope in bringing women's specific needs to light is that it reveals the impact our social world has on the experience of neurodiversity. This is an opportunity to think about how we actually support people with divergent needs in general. How can we respond *without* assuming that these needs make them deficient? Does this require a diagnosis? And, if it does, can we reconcile this with a response that is creative, rather than merely corrective? Can we support autistic women – and therefore all autistic people, perhaps even all neurodivergent people – in the aspects of their experience they enjoy, rather than simply mitigating 'abnormal' behaviour?

Who better to ask what real progress would look like, than autistic people themselves.

Non-medical advocacy has played a major role in shaping research agendas and public understanding of autism, perhaps more so than any DSM 'disorder'. In fact, many of the parent-led movements that have shaped the public awareness and research agendas for a host of conditions, like schizophrenia and depression, emerged as a result of the impetus generated around autism. *Self-advocacy*, on the other hand, has taken longer to gain momentum. To get their voices heard, autistic people built on the forums and blueprints laid by parent advocates, but claimed them to drive attention to the priorities that they, as autistic people, could uniquely identify. This meant challenging the preconceptions of scientists and even well-intentioned parents. It also meant challenging a central tenet of the parent-advocacy movement that had emerged through a history of turning to particular scientific authorities to bolster its demands for better support, the idea that autism needed to be 'cured'.

The rise of the internet has facilitated connection, advocacy and resource sharing, giving autistic people new ways to connect online.[21] In 1996, one of the first mailing lists, founded by Martijn Dekker, an autistic person based in the Netherlands, was launched – The Independent Living on the Autistic Spectrum (InLv).[22] While researchers were doubling down on autism as primarily a male issue, women in InLv discussions were already raising the factors[23] that were preventing them from getting diagnosed.[24] These women emphasised the role of socialisation in shaping the way their autistic traits manifested, and the degree of pressure they experienced to behave like 'normal' women, in their social lives, and in therapy.

The InLv list allowed the autistic people posting to flag the difficulties that mattered *to them*, rather than to parents or professionals. While the symptoms named in the classic 'triad' of behaviours used to diagnose autism – repetitive behaviours, differences in communication style, form and frequency, or desire for sameness – might be difficult for parents or others to understand and make sense of, the issues autistic people highlighted revolved primarily around sensual-perceptual differences (which may very well underly many of the behaviours medical research has pathologised), auditory processing, multitasking, face-blindness (prosopagnosia), and difficulties with time-keeping and completing projects (inertia), as well as strengths in focus on details and interests, and key differences in communication style.[25]

Self-advocacy brought to light issues that matter to the daily lived experience of autistic people themselves. In doing so, it highlighted the ways in which anyone presenting with non-'classic' autism symptoms often failed to get diagnosed. There are lots of people who fall outside diagnostic paradigms whose autism does not manifest in a typical way. Attention to women's exclusion helps to highlight the problem of exclusion in general, and so, the inadequacy of a treatment focused on, as Dekker writes, 'ways to make their autistic children indistinguishable from their peers, if not curing them altogether.'[26]

The 1993 essay *Don't Mourn for Us*,[27] written by the autism rights-activist Jim Sinclair, emerged from the self-advocacy movement, and is considered to be a founding document of the online autism community and culture. It became a touchstone, providing a counter-narrative to the 'tragedy model' of autism. In it, Sinclair gave the autistic community a manifesto, aimed at parents and engaged directly with the pervasive narrative of 'mourning' for the normal child they had expected, which typical parent literature, published by major charities, often still discusses as an expected stage of adjustment.[28] Instead, it asked parents and professionals to value autistic people as and how they are. Sinclair acknowledged the challenges their children's divergence presented to parents, but he invited the possibilities that acceptance and curiosity would bring: 'Push for the things your expectations tell you are normal, and you'll find frustration, disappointment, resentment, maybe even rage and hatred. Approach respectfully, without preconceptions, and with openness to learning new things, and you'll find a world you could never have imagined.'[29] Over thirty years later, many psychiatrists have yet to take heed of this important directive.

Another key figure, largely recognised as popularising the term 'neurodiversity', is Judy Singer, a social scientist who places herself on the autistic spectrum, and used the term in her sociology undergraduate thesis in 1997. In doing so, she was taking inspiration from the InLv discussions she had joined.[30]

Neurodiversity draws on a social model of disability and separates the impairment (the individual effect of loss or lack of a limb, function, or mechanism of the body) from disability, which the disability rights movement has defined as disadvantage, restriction, or oppression of people with impairments caused by physical and institutional barriers to access, social exclusion, and stigma. In this view, the difficulties of a particular form of neurodivergence are not ignored – a person may need particular forms of support, but it is the failure of the world to meet their needs that disables them. Their divergence from the perceived 'norm' is not, as Sinclair argued, the problem to be fixed – divergence is a given of human existence. It is the world that imposes barriers and norms that can and should change.

It is easy to think this view only applies to conditions that are not necessarily obviously distressing in and of themselves. But we have to remember that autism was initially viewed this way. Even for people with higher levels of autism, who may experience seizures, might find aspects of their experience distressing in and of themselves, the care structure and social response will make their experience easier or harder. The same could be said for experiences like depression or psychosis. In this view is a model for a primarily social response to mental diversity, whether it is painful or not. Medication or an aim of a cure may or may not be helpful to a person, but adequate social support and an accepting environment will always be key.

Neurodiversity offers a different research agenda for autistic women, too. Awareness that women have autism and research that attempts to explain how their autism differs cognitively may be interesting, but will only go so far. Some of the findings on cognition and autism, or insights that help diagnose and potentially provide better practical support, might yet prove to be helpful. Similarly, some autistic people find medical treatments, like drugs, helpful, although these treat accompanying issues, like anxiety and depression, not autism itself. But it remains rare for medical research to interrogate the concept of 'normal' behaviour, or the 'normal' human brain, and until it does, neuroscience research will continue to reinforce a difference that implies that the abnormal, autistic mind, needs to be cured.

Much of the ongoing autism advocacy also remains more concerned with mitigating the struggles of parents, than that of the autistic people themselves in a world that expects conformity, rather than offering accommodations. While similar groups founded by parents of children with other developmental disabilities, like the National Down Syndrome Congress and The Arc, have long moved past lobbying for 'cures', and towards acceptance and facilitating neurodiversity in institutions, largely as a result of self-advocacy, the largest force in the autism field, Autism

Speaks, has only two autistic board members at the time of writing, and have yet to fund any substantive autistic-led initiatives. Indeed, they adopt a rhetoric that is generally hostile to autistic people.[31] Rather than funding or advocating for the service improvements and support autistic children and adults need to lead successful and more independent lives, Autism Speaks has poured most of its funding into research that critics say have eugenic goals, because it seems to pose as its ideal the extermination of autistic people altogether.[32] Its publicity material over the years has sent a similar message. Some particularly heinous examples include the 'I Am Autism' ad, posted in 2009, removed shortly after. The ad uses melodramatic language to evoke a personification of autism as a vague hybrid of a stalker, murderer and epidemic. 'I know where you live', 'I work faster than paediatric AIDS, cancer, and diabetes combined', 'You are scared and you should be', are some of its most memorable quotes.[33] Then there is the 2006 documentary *Autism Every Day*, spotlighting parents who hate their autistic children. One interview in particular stands out, where a mother talks about wanting to kill her child by driving off a bridge. Even having recently updated its website to be less parent-centric, and to remove some of its most egregious statements about the supposed tragedy that is autism, the rhetoric seems tokenistic when its board continues to consist mainly of parents, not autistic people, and when its research and treatment goals still seem to emphasise making autism go away.

Autism Speaks remains the world's largest independent funding body of autism research,[34] and influences the priorities of the largest funder, the US Government, through strategic lobbying, but also employs researchers in Europe and Asia, especially in countries where funding is difficult to get, and is actively seeking to expand outside of the US.[35] It has a significant influence on the direction autism research takes. As a result, the vast majority of research funded is concerned with what causes autism and how it should be 'treated', rather than how to improve individual outcomes through education, public policy, combating discrimination, and improving support for autistic people and their families.[36] Other major autism organisations in the US have focused similarly on state-by-state battles to ensure that health insurance covers 'treatments', such as applied behaviour analysis (ABA), a therapy that tackles what is deemed to be problematic behaviour, and encourages socially adaptive behaviour.[37] Operant conditioning, used in ABA, is the practice of rewarding desired actions and punishing unwanted actions. It is used on animals and humans and has a history of using shocks as punishment. Beyond the obvious – that this is dehumanising – the technique is purely behavioural. It is intended to get people behaving in line with the 'norm'.

The very widespread and medicalised view of autism today, in which autism is a disorder to be treated rather than an instance of diversity to be accommodated, can be explained in part by the collaboration between parent advocates and doctors in its history. We saw how the parents of schizophrenic children in the 1970s found comfort in the biological explanations that offered an alternative to the parent-blaming culture fuelled by psychoanalysis. Biology offered reprieve, but it was also a vessel for authoritative, yet largely unproven and greatly inflated, promises of cures. Parent advocates united with scientists to push for research that shifted blame from bad parenting to the innate biological defect, and this suited scientists who were interested in procuring funding for their medical research. When the

American Congress allocated $40 million to the National Institute of Mental Health (NIMH) mostly for the support of schizophrenia research in 1985, the organisation credited the National Alliance on Mental Illness (NAMI) for its lobbying efforts for the decision.[38] Parents went on to set up private charities that funded new research into the biological understanding of mental disease, and this continues to be a common funding source today.

We cannot, of course, deny the necessity of parent-advocacy when it emerged; a time when it was believed that autistic children were irrevocably broken (by their parents), making support services futile. Parents saw the need for structural support and care, and so they looked where they could to get their movement off the ground. Yet approval from and collaboration with doctors was a driving force in the parent-advocacy movement, and it promoted a particular, medical view of autism that is not necessarily helpful to autistic people themselves. Parents' struggle nor their important work should be minimised, but there remains the fact of that eerie silence in this history of advocacy that should make all of us uncomfortable: the absence of the autistic people themselves.

The history of parent-advocacy helps explain the heightened public awareness around autism in recent years, and the progress that has been made in drawing attention to this way of experiencing the world. Their work has helped make autism a public, rather than parental, issue. Their work has boosted research, some of which has been helpful in supporting autistic people, and that is undeniable progress. Yet the very specific medical focus that has emerged through this campaigning also explains why autistic people have had much work to do, particularly in more recent decades, in changing the framing of autism from a disorder to be cured, to a way of being that requires social change, and structural, individualised support.

A different science

Dr Mitzi Waltz is a disability studies scholar who has worked in autism studies for over thirty years, first as a parent advocate and then as a researcher in the US, then the UK, and now in the Netherlands. She has participated in and observed the changing tone and focus of the scholarship and activism over that time. When we spoke, I was most struck by her humane insight. She told me that, for a while at least, she thought things were moving in the right direction. But, she lamented, 'the millions of dollars poured into the biomedical system in the US changed all that.' That 2006 investment reanimated biomedical research into autism, reflecting the idea, once again, that this was a condition to 'treat' or 'cure'.

Waltz went on to explain: 'We don't assume that for intellectual disability – we assume it's education and care we need, but we don't try to change the disability itself.' Autism was, in her words, 're-pathologised'. That influence has pushed into Europe and Asia, via the financial flows of pharmaceutical and genetic data companies, undoing much of the progress that researchers and advocates made.

Autistic people continue to ask questions about the purpose and results of autism research, proving repeatedly how it is crucial to involve the people affected in the scientific studies that try to understand them. The Canadian autistic woman and researcher Michelle Dawson has shown how research findings linked to autism are generally presented as abnormal or negative – even when autistic subjects perform better than non-autistic subjects on a task.[39] Research and research guidance predicated on relative strengths in autism is emerging, but is overshadowed by the much larger body of deficit-focused work. Similarly, much of the academic research untangling gender nonconformity and autism today, and providing gender-sensitive resources, continues to come from people with lived experience of autism. This research is often translated into practical initiatives and guides, such as Robyn Stuart's *Autism-Friendly Guide to Periods*, or Wenn Lawson's *The Autistic Trans Guide to Life*.

A shift towards an approach based on improved quality of life, rather than reaffirming deficits or difference, is more likely to actually improve the lives of autistic people. In 2010, Scott Michael Robertson, another autistic researcher, at Penn State University, called for a shift in autism research towards improving quality of life.[40] He asked researchers to collaborate with autistic people, to devise studies that aimed to better understand how autistic people learn and develop, and then to provide the services and support they need. He posited this as an alternative to the deficit model of autism that is used to justify prenatal testing and abortion of potentially affected foetuses, or invasive treatments aimed at wiping out all features associated with autism, whether or not these may have beneficial aspects.

In some countries, including the US, prenatal testing is available to parents who already have an autistic child, allowing them to terminate a pregnancy if a child is predicted to be on the spectrum.[41] The extent to which autism is defined by genes remains a mystery. Yet research has shown that if a family has one autistic child, the likelihood of a future child being autistic is as high as 25 per cent.[42] In an ableist culture, these statistics become the rationale for developing effective tests to detect some mutations associated with autism in foetuses. Diagnostic tests are still far from definitive; researchers are still trying to understand how any given mutation might lead to autism, and in any case, most autism is polygenically inherited, meaning there are many genes contributing to it. Even if two people carry the same genetic variant, one may have a very severe syndrome and the other much milder – or no syndrome at all.[43] Tests can only detect some variants linked to autism, and even then, the crucial, determining factor in how these genes will translate into a person and a life lived are completely ignored. The prenatal tests used for autism are largely developed by commercial companies and each lab screens for its own set of autism genes and draws often very speculative conclusions. Yet studies that aim to find accurate tests continue to sprout up.[44] The hope of prenatal testing is alive and well. Whatever the ethical regulation around these tests may turn out to be (if there is any), the intention behind pre-natal testing is to terminate suspected autistic (and so, less desirable) children. This is a form of modern-day eugenics. The testing also ignores the fact that social support structures determine whether an autistic person will live a fulfilling life or not. These studies then also continue to reinforce the myth of a biological root we have seen with schizophrenia, that autism is a problem 'within' the person, as a biological problem in them, rather than one that exists in society.

Of course, targeting social support structures will require much more radical overhaul than a new drug. We have seen how the research pipeline in psychiatry is increasingly financially driven. In the area of autism, too, pharmaceutical companies have worked with the non-profit Autism Speaks and university-based researchers with an eye to developing drugs that might address 'autistic symptoms'.[45] This is the same drive to 'treat' autism we saw expressed in the ABA therapy. It is equally reflected in the drive to find new drugs to make autism go away.

Another theory about how autism develops draws on the concept of neuroinflammation.[46] If neuroinflammation is involved in autism, this could potentially yield some fairly straightforward drug treatments involving anti-inflammatories to 'treat' autism (read: make it disappear).[47] Researchers have landed on a potential role for extreme forms of brain inflammation in some cases of autism. One piece of (not yet published) research showed how brain inflammation in children was linked to autism, and, the researchers argue, other 'neurological disorders' like schizophrenia.[48] It has to be noted that this study concerned largely children who had died from the condition that caused inflammation, so this was not a typical autism population by any means. Nonetheless, there are precedents for this link between neuroinflammation and autism. The last major epidemic for rubella, a viral infection that causes a spotty rash and a fever, before the vaccine became available in 1969, coincided with a spike in autism cases, as well as causing many children to go deaf, blind, and/or experiencing other birth defects.[49] Rubella can cause encephalitis, where the brain becomes inflamed, but these cases were only related to children exposed to the disease during gestation.[50] All in all, inflammation might be a factor in some cases of autism, but only in rare, severe cases of inflammation that would require medical treatment for a whole range of health effects. This means that, technically, what we are describing is not autism according to the DSM-5 definition, but that the term is used to describe a comparable experience. Encephalitis can cause symptoms that in the absence of illness might be attributed to autism, such as sensory sensitivity, behavioural changes, aphasia and apraxia of speech.[51] This shows us again how the categories of the DSM, which define mental disorders as categories of symptoms, often miss the meaning of these experiences to people; it isn't helpful to relegate autistic people and people with encephalitis to the same category, because it doesn't help psychiatrists or mental health professionals meet people and their needs.

Of course, none of this needs to imply that because autism might in some exceptional cases be linked to a biological inflammation, that the way of experiencing what we call autism is in itself pathological. It does not follow that autism itself needs to be 'cured'. But within a culture primed for a medical response to mental variation, findings like these easily become arguments for a cure.

A quick Google search for neuroinflammation and autism will turn up the following advice right at the top of the page: 'Good nutritional guidance and supplementation of vitamins, minerals, essential fatty acids and antioxidants is an integral part of re-regulating cellular function and reduction of inflammation in the body'. Dr Waltz described to me how this is just the tip of the iceberg of a whole system of labs, predominantly in the US, that promise to provide an extensive analysis of your autistic child's deficits, based on some kind of biological sample.[52] The 'treatment' in all cases is a range of purchasable products, often nutritional supplements. Tests have shown that customers will receive the same generic list regardless of what sample they send; a sample of hair from someone who isn't autistic, accompanied by application forms that simply state that the sample is from an autistic person, will yield the same treatment.[53] Many of these 'labs' also sell supplements or have interlocking director-ates with companies that do. This has been ongoing since the 1990s, with very little pushback from the FDA, or any other agency that should be checking. FDA funding, it's worth adding, is funded by a congress of which two-thirds of its former members go on to join lobbying industries. Commercial interests are once again driving the sale of harmful, phoney products.

And so, as women's autism is coming into the light and diagnosis is becoming more inclusive, it's important to remember that this newfound awareness still exists in a paradigm that promotes conformity and medical 'normal-ity' rather than social change and real improvement to the services and supports available. Awareness is not enough. The newfound visibility of autistic women, and autism generally, evident in recent media depictions and report-ing is hopeful, but real progress will come from acting on that newfound awareness. We need to ask what real work is being done to change the way we respond to autism and disability. We need to turn to the questions raised by dis-ability activists and autistic self-advocates to draw on the potential of autistic women to change the way psychiatry understands and responds to mental experiences currently deemed abnormal and pathological. Discussions about the cutting-edge science we currently value as a society con-flate medical and social progress.

A neurodiversity perspective suggests a different kind of relationship between psychiatrists and their patients. Women and girls have been excluded from autism research and support as a result of an expert-led paradigm; psychia-trists asking the questions, informed by their assumptions, to produce scientific knowledge about people. The most helpful support for women and girls with autism involves an understanding of their world, and involves talking to them; it involves studying and valuing the experience of individuals, rather than imposing a norm on them. In this, there are new principles for psychiatry as a whole; less profitable, perhaps, than neuroscience, but more helpful.

Appropriate support should factor in the difficulties identified by autistic people themselves, should be sensory-sensitivity-aware, and based on the forms of communication that work best for the person in question. It should be attuned to the traumas they may have experienced as women *and* as autistic people. It should also, of course, be reliable and accessible in terms of time, space and cost, lest we exclude people based on socioeconomic status. And the goals should be the goals set by the autistic people themselves, rather than those that aim to make people look and act 'normal'.

I spoke with Becky Choat, a project lead at the Scottish charity SWAN, which provides services and peer-support for autistic women and non-binary people. The organisation was formed around the question raised by its founder, Dr Catriona Stewart OBE, in her PhD and subsequent research: 'Where can we be what we are?' This is a very different question from what 'causes' autism, or 'how do we "cure" it?' The swan analogy in the name echoes that experience of many autistic women that we have seen, who learn to mask their autistic traits to meet societal expectations and fit into a neurotypical world. On the surface, these women 'may appear to glide effortlessly across the surface of life, whilst frantically paddling underneath just to stay afloat.'[54] Yet SWAN's aim is not to 'get behind the mask' of these women, to explain their 'true' nature in medical terms, but to provide the social connection, resources and peer support they need to lead more fulfilling lives. The charity recognises that women don't have a different form of autism to men but do experience unique *social* pressures that will present unique challenges to an autistic person, and requires different resources and support. It isn't cutting-edge science, it's actually incredibly obvious. We don't need to explain autism, we don't need scientific breakthroughs or miracle products; we just need to take people's needs at face value and respond accordingly. We give research orphans a home by moving away from deficits-based research and towards research that is useful to autistic people themselves.

Conclusion

The Other Side

'If a plant were wilting we wouldn't diagnose it with "wilting-plant-syndrome" – we would change its conditions.'[1]
Dr Sanah Ahsan

Throughout this book we've repeatedly encountered the limits of a solely medical approach to mental distress. We have seen how diagnoses are based on inconsistent research that vastly overstates the scientific certainty of these concepts, especially of their existence as diseases in our brains and genes. We have also seen how this scientific objectivity of authoritative manuals, in particular the DSM, masks historic and current prejudice encoded in diagnostic concepts in a way that perpetuates discrimination but also consolidates a knowledge base built on assumptions rather than growing scientific insight. We have seen how these labels in many cases feed a society-wide stigmatisation of human experiences which isolates people and, for many, exacerbates their distress, even while some find that labels bring clarity and validation. We have seen how the medical view of mental health decontextualises mental disorder, removing it from its social environment, and so hiding the political causes of mental distress that are inseparable from any biological effects these may have, and that also contain a whole host of social and political solutions to mental suffering that exist outside the individual. We have seen that the financial and political power vested in the current medical view has led governments and industries to push dubious solutions on people. We have seen how a lack of cultural humility has made many of psychiatry's practices oppressive.

For that reason, it isn't clear why a medical view should continue to sit at the centre of our mental healthcare system. At least not in its current form.

We've also seen throughout this book, glimmers of a different vision from survivors of trauma, advocates of neurodiversity, and psychiatrists alike. Critics fall on a spectrum of those who believe in total abolition of the medical view and believe that individuals should decide and shape their own care, to those who believe there is a more measured, and slightly different role for medicine to play, and those who think that medical diagnosis can be part of a non-oppressive view of mental health that destig-matises difference.

But there are common denominators connecting many of the suggestions for a better psychiatry and a better mental healthcare system.

Most suggestions for reform propose that we first of all base our systems on a new narrative. They agree that the biological narrative of mental distress needs to be replaced with one based on the growing evidence for social, political, cultural and other, non-biological, causes of mental distress. This doesn't necessarily mean doing away with biological explanations – as we've seen, biology does often play a role – but it does mean no longer posing biological factors as the *primary* mechanism in causing mental distress, and being transparent about the limited role medical treatments can play.

A new multi-factorial narrative of mental distress leads to a different care offering. Even the most effective remedy for the low moods we call depression, or the visions we call psychosis, won't give a person the safety, resources, agency, understanding of the impact of life experiences and ongoing connection that may all be variously needed to recover from a mental health crisis. And that 'variously' is key. If we acknowledge that mental suffering doesn't happen in a vacuum, then we also need to take into account the specificity of a person's situation and needs. This means we cannot rely on cookie-cutter solutions. Luckily, people are usually quite clear on the help they need. As we saw in the case of psychedelics, people find a range of rituals helpful when it comes to healing; the main determining factor is that they chose the ritual themselves. Mental healthcare, in this view, needs to be less about administering cures, and more about facilitating choice. This also means that the first choice a person makes, has to be whether they have anything to 'recover' from at all. Perhaps they do not want a treatment plan, perhaps they just want some modicum of support through a difficult time. Perhaps they don't want to change, and merely want to cope. Perhaps all they want is a prescription; this all needs to be possible. Mental disorder has too long been a mechanism for discrimination, defining norms imposed on people, rather than supporting people in building lives that work for them. Psychiatrists will need to support people in designing the help they need. This may also involve supporting them in accessing welfare, finding community, or accessing culturally embedded resources that speak to the way people themselves make sense of their mental distress.[2]

In short, this new system is about fostering environments, rather than curing people. If we want to develop mental healthcare systems that respond seriously to the proven social determinants of mental health, we need to base them on a non-medical question. Not 'How do we cure people?' but instead: 'How can we foster environments that allow people to live their own, unique, fulfilling lives?' We need to return to Dr Catriona Stewart of SWAN's question for autistic women: 'Where can we be what we are?'

This approach is not utopian, but it will require radical reform. Jim van Os, cited in other chapters of this book, is part of the group of psychiatrists and mental healthcare consultants piloting, in various regions of the Netherlands, this exact modular approach that offers people a choice in their path to recovery. Speaking to me about the Dutch trials, van Os told me: 'The evidence shows that if you give people a meaningful ritual for change, it doesn't matter what it is. They will engage with it and improve, as long as it's compatible with their worldview and how they are.'

The Dutch mental healthcare trial enacts this principle. 'We foresee a large offering of group therapies depending on what the person wants', van Os told me in no uncertain terms, 'so if you say, "I feel depressed right now, I want to do meditation," then we refer you to a group for meditation. If you say, "I've been traumatised, I want to do a trauma-focused group approach," you can do that, you can do EDMR groups. If you say, "I want to work with a shamanistic ritual to help my mental suffering" then we have qualified people doing that.'

Some psychiatrists may shiver at the prospect of such a widely accommodating system. They may argue that we need to distinguish in the debates about what constitutes good mental healthcare, between the mild anxiety and depression which, many claim, are increasingly taken up (especially by young people) to pathologise normal human experience. This trend is clogging up mental healthcare systems, they argue, preventing people with more serious cases of acute psychosis or autistic seizures to access support. I agree that we need to ensure people get the support they need. But all the psychiatric diagnoses are connected by the same problem of an overmedicalisation of mental experience. Reforming our mental healthcare systems to make them multi-modal, not just medical, will, eventually, take pressure off an overstrained medical system that won't ever meet the diversity of needs currently, inappropriately, funnelled through the same services.

To make such an individualised approach to mental healthcare possible, will require several, further, shifts. It will rely, in very practical terms, on the right infrastructure, which will be built on new types of relationships. Psychiatrists will have to collaborate with various service providers, currently fragmented, to ensure people don't fall between the cracks. Psychiatrists can take a leading role in coordinating this care ecosystem. Some suggest that they would need to work as public health practitioners, rather than medical subspecialists. They would have to get good at building alliances and collaborating with colleagues from different specialities, as well as sectors beyond health, like the social care sector, or welfare, education and justice. [3]

In a non-medical system, psychiatrists' roles wouldn't be reduced, but expanded, beyond diagnosing and prescribing medication. They could still deal with medication but would need to be clear that treating a person's biology is a relatively superficial way of tackling a much broader problem that extends beyond their body or even the individual. They would have to explain that they can use drugs to manage symptoms for a short while, and, in addition, will need to be transparent about the side effects, and active in helping clients manage withdrawal from the drugs. Psychiatrists in this system would still be experts on medication, as they are today, but might, somewhat paradoxically, be more involved in getting people off drugs, than on them.[4] But this would be just part of their role. Becoming expert coordinators may prove to be a more likely way of maintaining psychiatry's status in the mental health field, rather than clinging to a medical model that is increasingly recognised as only a partial response to mental distress.[5]

Psychiatrists may, equally, still use the language of diagnosis, but in a much more limited way. Perhaps they'll use broad diagnostic categories to describe a person's mental experience; a passing state of depression or anxiety, rather than an inherent disorder. But it has to be said that psychiatrists can do their job without diagnosis, as we have seen; the concept of formulation, for example, is about agreeing on an explanation of a person's current mental experience without the need for a label. As ever, we need to think carefully about the implications of such a change for people who currently gain clarity and support through these diagnoses.

Ultimately, the language psychiatrists use will undoubtedly change, because it will be shaped by a very different principle. It won't reflect the latest classifications in manuals, so much as what helps people make sense of their experience in order to shape their own support. The words they choose will be in service of the supportive relationship they are trying to build with the people they used to know as patients. The new psychiatry will be an exercise in advanced relationship-building. Not the cutting-edge science of new drugs or brain scans, but intricate, supportive networks of alliances for care. So many studies support the finding that it is the therapeutic alliance, the feeling that someone gets that they are supported, that matters as much, or more, than any medication or treatment a person receives to any improvements they experience. [6] We have also already seen how, in the cases where psychiatrists underwent peer support training, they found greater professional satisfaction in relationships based on a shared humanity, rather than differential expertise.

Making the relationship rather than medical treatment the primary focus for the psychiatrist also changes the role of control in psychiatric care. Any imposition against a person's will, any assumption to know what is best for them, will undermine their collaborative, equal relationship. This is not to turn a blind eye to cases of, for example, psychopathy or ASPD that affect communities. Nor is it to disregard the range in people's capacities for self-directed support, depending on the intensity of their mental experience or distress. It is only to sever the link between mental distress and disorder, or, at its extreme, criminality. Psychiatrists will have to reverse the assumption that people in distress are risky, and to assume, instead, that, given the right support, they can continue to make their own decisions about their support.

Emphasising collaboration, though, also doesn't necessarily mean doing away with involuntary containment altogether. We have seen that there are models for care that support individuals in developing a crisis plan, that grants permission to the caregiver to restrict their freedom in the case of an emergency. Once a relationship is established, people will trust the person caring for them, even

during periods of extreme tension or confusion, to imple-
ment periods of confinement or medication, with an eye
to keeping them safe until they are ready to take the reins
again.[7] This is not naïve. As we have seen, it has worked in
prisons, among peer-networks, and in psychiatric hospitals. It just needs staff training, enough time, resourcing
and adequate management.

  All of this, of course, relies on adequate funding going
into the existing alternatives to psychiatric care that
already exist everywhere; so much essential care happens in
siloed and underfunded pockets. As much as the scientific
narrative makes us believe knowledge is progress, progress
in this case is simply drawing on the wealth of experience that already exists, and resourcing and connecting
these in an overarching infrastructure. This may also take
some of the pressure off mainstream services. As we have
seen, services are strained, GPs often struggle to get their
patients admitted to psychiatric care, and patients are left
to languish once they leave. We need to invest, first and
foremost, in creating the conditions for person-centred
care and coordinated support. Governments talk increasingly of funding mental healthcare, but pumping money
into a broken system won't work. We need to reform
and revise the principles underlying the system, invest
in restructuring and training, and then provide ongoing
financial support. Assumptions that people cannot heal
in communities are nothing more than laissez-faire justifications for the current distribution of power. People can
heal in community; examples like Trieste are evidence of
that. The Trieste model has drastically reduced the need
for hospitalisation since it was established. It only works,
though, because it is a well-supported and coordinated
web of services, integrated within the wider community,

to provide robust healing environments to support people in living their lives on their own terms.

This reminds us that without an adequate social structure to support a system, any attempt at mental healthcare reform will fall flat. This is also true for the wider social context – no mental healthcare system will be able to accommodate the influx of people in crisis if social conditions don't improve. Mental healthcare systems are in themselves not solutions to social neglect. Without social change to tackle the disparities and remove the obstacles that people face at various intersections of oppression, even the most inclusive mental health system will be entirely tokenistic. To recognise the social factors that cause mental distress means tackling mental health not just as a public health issue but a social justice issue. Governments need to enact human values aimed at equitable quality of life. Without basic rights, mental health is meaningless.

And yet, mental healthcare reform could be revolutionary. Mental suffering sediments and consolidates socio-economic disparity. A supportive mental health system is a crucial cornerstone of an inclusive society. And we have a map that can take us there.

To put people at the heart of mental healthcare will involve many professions and services working together. Psychiatry has a major part to play, given the powerful role it plays in shaping government agendas, as well as our language and understanding of mental health today. For reform to work, psychiatry will have to play a new and different role. The profession will have to revise its slogans. It will have to stop selling cures and, instead, work to support a suitable environment for people to be well. This is the work of removing obstacles to wellbeing. It will need to stop asserting its medical expertise and take up its place in a collaborative effort with other services, on local, national and global levels to deliver individualised support. This is the work of facilitating choice. To turn to the garden and trust the plants' ability to grow.

Notes

Introduction – Psychiatry and Society: A Mental Health Tragedy

1 D. Richter, A. Wall, A. Bruen, R. Whittington, 'Is the global prevalence rate of adult mental illness increasing? Systematic review and meta-analysis', *Acta Psychiatrica Scandinavica*, 140 (2019), pp. 393–407; https://www.theguardian.com/society/2019/jun/03/mental-illness-is-there-really-a-global-epidemic

2 'World mental health report', *World Health Organisation*, 2022.

3 Deb Gordon, 'Mental Health Drug Usage Rose in 2021, But Not All Pharmacy Costs Did, New Report Shows', *Forbes*, October 9, 2022.

4 Dainius Pūras, 'Report of the Special Rapporteur on the Right of Everyone to the Enjoyment of the Highest Attainable Standard of Physical and Mental Health', *UN Doc* A/HRC/44/48 ('Pūras Report 44/48') (15 April 2020); Yvette Maker & Bernadette McSherry, 'Human rights and the social determinants of mental health: fostering interdisciplinary research collaboration', *Psychiatry, Psychology and Law*, (19 Sep 2023) DOI: 10.1080/13218719.2023.2243297.

5 'Mental health, human rights and legislation: guidance and practice', *World Health Organisation*, October 9, 2023.

6 Annabel Rackham, 'Nearly half a million more adults on antidepressants in England', *BBC News*, July 9 2023.

7 Ruth Brauer et al., 'Psychotropic medicine consumption in 65 countries and regions, 2008–19: a longitudinal study', *The Lancet*, 8, no. 12 (2021): 1071–1082. doi.org/10.1016/S2215-0366(21)00292-3.

8 E. Dumas-Mallet and F. Gonon, 'Messaging in biological psychiatry: misrepresentations, their causes, and potential consequences', *Harvard Review Psychiatry*, 28, no. 6 (2020): 395–403. doi.org/10.1097/HRP.0000000000000276.

9 I. W. Browne, 'American psychiatry and the cult of psychoanalysis', *J. Ir. Med. Assoc.* 1964. qtd. in Jim van Os, Sinan Guloksuz, 'Schizophrenia as a symptom of psychiatry's reluctance to enter the

moral era of medicine,' *Schizophrenia Research*, 242, (2022): 138–140. doi.org/10.1016/j.schres.2021.12.017.

10 'How Often Does Sexual Assault Occur in the United States?' *RAINN* (2024).

11 S. Scott and S. McManus, 'Hidden Hurt. Violence, abuse and disadvantage in the lives of women', *Agenda* (2016).

12 'Mental Health Inequalities', *Centre for Mental Health*, 2020; P. Mainali, F. Motiwala, C. Trivedi, R. Vadukapuram, Z. Mansuri, S. Jain, 'Sexual Abuse and Its Impact on Suicidal Ideation and Attempts and Psychiatric Illness in Children and Adolescents With Post-traumatic Stress Disorder', *Prim Care Companion CNS Disord*, 17;25(1):22m03239 (2023). doi: 10.4088/PCC.22m03239. PMID: 36705981.

13 'Mental Health Inequalities', *Centre for Mental Health*, 2020.

14 'More than 4 in 10 U.S. Adults Who Needed Substance Use and Mental Health Care Did Not Get Treatment', *National Council for Mental Wellbeing*, 2021.

15 'Mental Health Inequalities', *Centre for Mental Health*, 2020.

16 Olympia L. K. Campbell, David Bann, Praveetha Patalay, 'The gender gap in adolescent mental health: A cross-national investigation of 566,829 adolescents across 73 countries', *SSM – population health*, volume 13 (2021). doi.org/10.1016/j. ssmph.2021.100742; Yu, Shoukai, 'Uncovering the hidden impacts of inequality on mental health: a global study,' *Translational psychiatry*, vol. 8,1 98 (2018) doi:10.1038/s41398-018-0148-0.

17 'Mental Health Disparities: Women's Mental Health', American Psychiatric Association, 2017.

18 Anila M. D'Mello et al, 'Exclusion of females in autism research: Empirical evidence for a 'leaky' recruitment-to-research pipeline', *Autism research : official journal of the International Society for Autism Research* vol. 15,10 (2022): 1929–1940. doi:10.1002/aur.2795.

19 R. McCrossin, 'Finding the True Number of Females with Autistic Spectrum Disorder by Estimating the Biases in Initial Recognition and Clinical Diagnosis', *Children* (Basel), 9(2):272 (2022) doi: 10.3390/children9020272. PMID: 35204992; PMCID: PMC8870038.

1: Hysteria, PTSD and the Birth of Psychiatry

1 T. J. Torrico, J. H. French, S. P. Aslam, et al, 'Histrionic Personality Disorder' in *Treasure Island* (FL: StatPearls Publishing, 2024).

2 George Didi-Huberman, *Invention of Hysteria: Charcot and the*

Photographic Iconography of the Salpêtrière (Cambridge, MA: MIT Press, 2004).

3   Barry Stephenson 'Charcot's Theatre of Hysteria', *Journal of Ritual Studies*, vol. 15, no. 1 (2001), pp. 27–37.

4   Sander Gilman, *Seeing the Insane* (New York: John Wiley and Sons, 1982).

5   Appignanesi, p. 148.

6   *Iconographie photographique de la Salpêtrière*, 1876, in Appignanesi, p. 149.

7   Appignanesi, p. 149.

8   Ibid, p. 150.

9   Ibid, p. 149.

10 Ibid.

11 Ibid, p. 149–152.

12 Ibid.

13 Ibid, 2008, p.149–152.

14 Lisa Appignanesi, *Mad, Bad and Sad* (Virago, 2008) p. 147.

15 M. S. Micale, 'Hysteria and its Historiography: A Review of Past and Present Writings (II)', *History of Science*, 27(4) (1989) pp.319–351. doi. org/10.1177/007327538902700401.

16 Appignanesi, p. 165.

17 Hippolyte Bernheim, 'Hypnotisme et suggestion: Doctrine de la Salpêtrière et doctrine de Nancy', *Le Temps* (supplement) (January 29, 1891): 1–2, in Harrington, p. 21.

18 Harrington, 2019, p. 23.

19 Ibid.

20 Herman, *Trauma and Recovery*, 1992, p. 19.

21 Ibid.

22 Cecily Devereux, 'Hysteria, Feminism, and Gender Revisited: The Case of the Second Wave', *ESC* 40.1 (2014), p. 24.

23 Sigmund Freud, *Female Sexuality. The Standard Edition of the Complete Psychological Works of Sigmund Freud,' Volume XXI (1927 –1931): The Future of an Illusion, Civilization and its Discontents, and Other Works*, 227 (1931), in Cecily Devereux, 'Hysteria, Feminism, and Gender Revisited: The Case of the Second Wave', *ESC* 40.1 (2014), pp. 19–45.

24 General Remarks on Hysterical Attacks, S. Freud, *Female Sexuality. The Standard Edition of the Complete Psychological Works of Sigmund Freud, Volume XXI (1927- 1931): The Future of an Illusion, Civilization and its Discontents, and Other Works*, 124 (1931), in Devereux, p. 24.

25 Cecily Devereux, 'Hysteria, Feminism, and Gender Revisited: The Case of the Second Wave', *ESC* 40.1 (March 2014), p. 24.

26 Ibid, pp. 19–45.

27 Sigmund Freud, *The History of the Psychoanalytic Movement* (New York: Nervous and Mental Disease Pub. Co., 1917)

28 Ibid.

29 Charles S. Myers, 'A contribution to the study of shell shock: being an account of three cases of loss of memory, vision, smell, and taste, admitted into the Duchess of Westminster's War Hospital, Le Touquet', *The Lancet*, 1915.

30 Ibid.

31 Harrington, 2019, p. 26.

32 Charles S. Myers, 'A Final Contribution THE STUDY OF SHELL SHOCK.1: BEING A CONSIDERATION OF UNSETTLED POINTS NEEDING INVESTIGATION,' *The Lancet*, Volume 193, Issue 4976, 1919, Pages 51–54.

33 Harrington, 2019, p. 27.

34 A. Kardiner & H. Spiegel, *War, stress, and neurotic illness* (Rev. ed.) (New York: Hoeber, 1947), p. 1.

35 G. C. Lasiuk, RN, MN, CPMHN (C), and K. M. Hegadoren, RN, PhD, 'Post-traumatic Stress Disorder Part I: Historical Development of the Concept', *Perspectives in Psychiatric Care* vol. 42, No. 1 (2006); P. Birmes, L. Hatton, A. Brunet and L. Schmitt, 'Early historical literature for post-traumatic symptomatology', *Stress and Health*, *19*(1) (2003)17–26; C. Moreau and S. Zisook, 'Rationale for post-traumatic stress spectrum disorder', *Psychiatric Clinics of North America*, 25(4) (2002), pp. 775 –790.

36 B. A. Van der Kolk and A. McFarlane, 'The black hole of trauma,' in B. A. Van der Kolk, A. McFarlane, & L. Weisaeth (Eds.), *Traumatic stress: The effects of overwhelming experience on mind, body, and society* (New York: Guilford Press, 1996), p. 48, qtd. in Lasiuk and Hegadoren, 2006.

37 Lasiuk and Hegadoren, 2006, p. 15.

38 Tracey Loughran, 'A Crisis of Masculinity? Re-writing the History of Shell-shock and Gender in First World War Britain', *History Compass*, Volume 11, Issue 9 (2013), pp. 727–738; M. Higgonet and P. Higgonet, 'The Double Helix,' in M. Higgonet, J. Jenson, S. Michel and M. C. Weisz (eds.), *Behind the Lines: Gender and the Two World Wars* (New Haven and London: Yale University Press, 1987), pp. 31–47.

39 Lasiuk and Hegadoren, 2006, p. 18; D. H. Marlowe, *Psychological and psychosocial consequences of combat and deployment with special emphasis on the Gulf War* (2000) Retrieved January 27, 2006, from www.gulflink.osd.mil/ library/randrep/marlowe_paper/index.html

40 Lasiuk and Hegadoren, 2006, p.18

41 G. C. Lasiuk, RN, MN, CPMHN (C), and K. M. Hegadoren, RN, PhD, 'Post-traumatic Stress Disorder Part I: Historical Development of the Concept', *Perspectives in Psychiatric Care* Vol. 42, No. 1 (2006); P. Birmes, L. Hatton, A. Brunet, & L. Schmitt, 'Early historical literature for post-traumatic symptomatology', *Stress and Health*, *19*(1) (2003), pp. 17–26.; C. Moreau, & S. Zisook, 'Rationale for post-traumatic stress spectrum disorder', *Psychiatric Clinics of North America*, 25(4) (2002), pp. 775 –790.

42 Lasiuk and Hegadoren, 2006, p. 13.

43 Miranda Olff, 'Sex and gender differences in post-traumatic stress disorder: an update', *European Journal of Psychotraumatology* vol. 8,sup4 1351204 (2017) doi:10.1080/20008198.2017.1351204; C. A. van der Meer, A. Bakker, A. S. Smit, S. van Buschbach, M. den Dekker, G. J. Westerveld, R. C. Hutter, B. P. Gersons, M. Olff, 'Gender and Age Differences in Trauma and PTSD Among Dutch Treatment-Seeking Police Officers', *J Nerv Ment Dis* 205(2) (2017), pp. 87–92. doi: 10.1097/NMD.0000000000000562. PMID: 27434192; Amy Novotney 'Women who experience trauma are twice as likely as men to develop PTSD. Here's why,' American Psychological Association (2023).

44 'Epidemiological Facts About PTSD National Center for Post Traumatic Stress Disorder', *A National Center for PTSD Fact Sheet*. Retrieved April 1, 2005 from www.ncptsd.va.gov/facts/general/ fs_epidemiological.html; Chivers-Wilson, Kaitlin A., 'Sexual assault and posttraumatic stress disorder: a review of the biological, psychological and sociological factors and treatments', *McGill journal of medicine: MJM : an international forum for the advancement of medical sciences by students* vol. 9,2 (2006): 111–8.

45 C. Barter, M. McCarry, D. Berridge and K. Evans, Partner exploitation and violence in teenage intimate relationships, NSPCC [Online] (2009).

46 'Domestic abuse victim characteristics, England and Wales: year ending March 2019', Office for National Statistics (2019).

47 Bethany Bran, 'Trauma and Women', *Psychiatric Clinics*, volume 26, issue 3 (2003), p. 759–779. doi.org/10.1016/S0193-953X(03)00034-0

48 R. C. Kessler, A. Sonnega, E. Bromet, M. Hughes, & C. B. Nelson, 'Post-traumatic stress disorder in the National Comorbidity Survey', *Archives of General Psychiatry*, 52(12) (1995), pp. 1048–1060.

49 Ibid.

50 K. M. Hegadoren, G. C. Lasiuk and N. J. Coupland, 'Post-traumatic Stress Disorder Part III: Health Effects of Interpersonal Violence Among Women', *Perspectives in Psychiatric Care* vol. 42, No. 3 (2006).

51 J. S. Chandan, T. Thomas, C. Bradbury-Jones, R. Russell, S. Bandyopadhyay, K. Nirantharakumar, J. Taylor, 'Female Survivors of Intimate Partner Violence and Risk of Depression, Anxiety and Serious Mental Illness', *British Journal of Psychiatry* (2019).

52 J. S. Chandan, T. Thomas, C. Bradbury-Jones, R. Russell, S. Bandyopadhyay, K. Nirantharakumar, J. Taylor, 'Female Survivors of Intimate Partner Violence and Risk of Depression, Anxiety and Serious Mental Illness', *British Journal of Psychiatry* (2019); L. M. Howard, 'Interpersonal violence and mental health: new findings and paradigms for enduring problems', *Soc Psychiatry Psychiatr Epidemiol* 58 (2023), pp. 1731–1734. doi.org/10.1007/s00127-023-02431-1; Manon E. Hauw, Mathieu Revranche, Viviane Kovess-Masfety, Mathilde M. Husky, 'Sexual and Nonsexual Interpersonal Violence, Psychiatric Disorders, and Mental Health Service Use', *Journal of Traumatic Stress* (2020) doi.org/10.1002/jts.22638.

53 J. Campbell, A. S. Jones, J. Dienemann, et al. 'Intimate Partner Violence and Physical Health Consequences', *Arch Intern Med.*162(10) (2002), pp. 1157–1163. doi:10.1001/archinte.162.10.1157

54 May Ellsberg et al, 'Intimate partner violence and women's physical and mental health in the WHO multi-country study on women's health and domestic violence: an observational study', *The Lancet*, VOLUME 371, ISSUE 9619 (2008), pp. 1165–1172. doi.org/10.1016/S0140-6736(08)60522-X; Tsuyuki, Kiyomi et al., 'Physiological Changes from Violence-Induced Stress and Trauma Enhance HIV Susceptibility Among Women', *Current HIV/AIDS reports* vol. 16,1 (2019): 57–65. doi:10.1007/s11904-019-00435-8; Katrina Nash et al., 'Exposure to Domestic Abuse and the Subsequent Development of Atopic Disease in Women', *The Journal of Allergy and Clinical Immunology*, VOLUME 11, ISSUE 6 (2023), pp. 1752–1756; J. Daniels, A. Aldous, M. Pyra, et al., 'Lifetime sexual violence exposure in women compromises systemic innate immune mediators associated

with HIV pathogenesis: A cross-sectional analysis', *Women's Health*
18 (2022) doi:10.1177/17455057221099486
55 J. L. Herman, *Trauma and recovery: The aftermath of violence – From domestic abuse to political terror.* (New York: Basic Books, 1992).
56 Ibid, p. 4.
57 M. Cloitre, 'ICD-11 complex post-traumatic stress disorder: Simplifying diagnosis in trauma populations', *The British Journal of Psychiatry*, 216(3) (2020), pp. 129–131. doi:10.1192/bjp.2020.43.
58 T. J. Torrico, J. H. French, S. P. Aslam, et al. 'Histrionic Personality Disorder', in *Treasure Island* (FL: StatPearls Publishing; 2024).
59 Nahathai Wongpakaran, Tinakon Wongpakaran, Vudhichai Boonyanaruthee, Manee Pinyopornpanish & Suthi Intaprasert, 'Comorbid personality disorders among patients with depression', *Neuropsychiatric Disease and Treatment*, 11 (2015), pp. 1091–1096, DOI: 10.2147/NDT.S82884; French JH, Shrestha S., 'Histrionic Personality Disorder', in *Treasure Island* (FL: StatPearls Publishing, 2023). PMID: 31194465.
60 J. Sprock, 'Gender-Typed Behavioral Examples of Histrionic Personality Disorder', *Journal of Psychopathology and Behavioral Assessment* 22, 107–122 (2000). doi.org/10.1023/A:1007514522708
61 S. O. Lilienfeld, C. Van Valkenburg, K. Larntz, H. S. Akiskal, 'The relationship of histrionic personality disorder to antisocial personality and somatization disorders', *Am J Psychiatry*, Jun;143(6) (1986), pp. 718–22.
62 E. E. Wheeler, E. Kosterina and L. Cosgrove, 'Diagnostic and Statistical Manual of Mental Disorders(DSM), Feminist Critiques of', in *The Wiley Blackwell Encyclopedia of Gender and Sexuality Studies* (eds. A. Wong, M. Wickramasinghe, r. hoogland and N.A. Naples), (2016).

2: A Billion-Dollar Industry

1 Anne Harrington, 'Mental Health's Stalled (Biological) Revolution: Its Origins, Aftermath & Future Opportunities', *Daedalus*; 152 (4) (2023), pp. 166–185.
2 'Report No. 1: Shock Therapy', *Group for the Advancement of Psychiatry*, (September 15, 1947).
3 Edward H. Thompson Jr. and William Doll, 'The Burden of Families Coping with the Mentally Ill: An Invisible Crisis', *Family Relations* 31 (3) (1982), pp. 379–388. doi.org/10.2307/584170; Phyllis Vine, *Families in Pain: Children, Siblings, Spouses, and Parents of the*

Mentally Ill Speak Out (New York: Pantheon Books, 1982); Anne Harrington, 'Mental Health's Stalled (Biological) Revolution: Its Origins, Aftermath & Future Opportunities', *Daedalus*; 152 (4) (2023), pp. 166–185.

4   Ronald Bayer, *Homosexuality and American Psychiatry: The Politics of Diagnosis* (Princeton, N.J.: Princeton University Press, 1981); Jack Drescher and Joseph P. Merlino, eds., *American Psychiatry and Homosexuality: An Oral History* (New York: Harrington Park Press, 2007).

5   Peter Sedgwick, *Psycho Politics: Laing, Foucault, Goffman, Szasz, and the Future of Mass Psychiatry* (New York: Harper & Row, 1982); Norman Dain, 'Antipsychiatry', in *American Psychiatry after World War II*, ed. Roy W. Menninger and John C. Nemiah (Washington, D.C.: American Psychiatric Press, 2000), pp. 277–342.

6   Anne Harrington, 'Mental Health's Stalled (Biological) Revolution: Its Origins, Aftermath & Future Opportunities', *Daedalus*; 152 (4) (2023), pp. 166–185.

7   Hannah S. Decker, *The Making of DSM-III: A Diagnostic Manual's Conquest of American Psychiatry* (New York: Oxford University Press, 2013).

8   A Compston, 'Decade of the brain', *Brain*, 128 (2005), pp. 1741–1742.

9   M Goldstein, 'Decade of the brain. An agenda for the nineties', *Western Journal of Medicine*, 161(3) (1994), p. 239.

10 Mark Dennis Robinson, 'The Market in Mind: How Financialization Is Shaping Neuroscience', *Translational Medicine and Innovation in Biotechnology* (MIT Press, Cambridge, Massachusetts and London, 2019) p. 40.

11 Edward G. Jones; Lorne M. Mendell, 'Assessing the Decade of the Brain', *Science*. 284 (5415) (1999), p. 739.

12 Ibid.

13 Ibid.

14 Ibid.

15 Ibid.

16 Professor of bioethics, Mark Dennis Robinson has argued that the translational restructuring of neuroscience was not even just simply an opportunistic response to a perceived economic opportunity, but a more deliberate response to a specific market need. A surge of international biotechnology markets emerged during the global economic crisis starting in 2004–2005, as universities underwent rapid transformation and increasing

privatisation, and as biopharmaceutical companies were struggling, exacerbated during this global financial down-turn. The translational shift wasn't just a strategy geared towards greater health innovation, nor the result of a burgeoning scientific knowledge-base. It was a financially driven, deliberate, restructuring.

17 Elias A. Zerhouni, 'Translational and Clinical Science: Time for a New Vision', *New England Journal of Medicine*, 1622 (2005) in Robinson, 2019, p. 3.

18 Mark Dennis Robinson, 2019, p. 3.

19 Robinson, 2019, p.ix.

20 Ibid.

21 Harrington, 2019, p. 250.

22 Ibid.

23 'Prozac Print Campaign,' *Marketing Campaign Case Studies*, (October 15, 2008); Jean Grow, Jin Park and Xiaogi Han, 'Your Life Is Waiting!: Symbolic Meanings in Direct-to-Consumer Antidepressant Advertising', *Journal of Communication Inquiry* 30, no. 2 (2006), pp. 163–88.

24 Harrington, 2019, p. 215.

25 A. V. Horwitz, 'DSM – I and DSM – II', *Encyclopedia of Clinical Psychology*, eds R. L. Cautin and S. O. Lilienfeld (2014), in Micha Frazer-Carroll, 2023, Mad World, p. 46.

26 Harrington, 2019, pp. 247–8.

27 'Psychiatric Drug Discovery on the Couch', *Nature Reviews Drug Discovery* 6, no.3 (2007), doi.org/10.1038/nrd2268

28 Anne Harrington, 'Mental Health's Stalled (Biological) Revolution: Its Origins, Aftermath & Future Opportunities', *Daedalus* 152 (4) (2023), pp. 166–185. doi: doi.org/10.1162/daed_a_02037

29 Harrington, 2019, p. 251.

30 Fluoxetine: Drug Usage Statistics, United States, 2013–2022, *ClinCalc*, 2022.

31 Harrington, 2019, pp. 208–216.

32 Ibid.

33 Ibid.

34 P. D. Kramer, *Listening to Prozac* (New York: Penguin, 1994), pp. 9, 21, in Harrington, 2021.

35 Kramer, 1994, p. 15.

36 M. Fisher, *Capitalist Realism: Is There No Alternative?* (Winchester, UK: Zero books, 2009).

37 Harrington, 2019, p. 213.

38 Ibid, p. 252.

39 Ibid, p. 253.

40 Ibid, p. 267.

41 Steven Hyman, interview by Anne Harrington, November 24, 2010.

42 Harrington, 2019, p. 255.

43 Bali Sunset, 'Social Anxiety Disorder Campaign', *Marketing Campaign Case Studies* (blog), March 28, 2009.

44 Harrington, 2019, pp. 255–257.

45 E.g. 'Study: Media Perpetuates Unsubstantiated Chemical Imbalance Theory of Depression', *Florida State University News* (March 3, 2008); Christopher M. France, Paul H. Lysaker and Ryan P. Robinson, 'The "Chemical Imbalance" Explanation for Depression: Origins, Lay Endorsement, and Clinical Implications', *Professional Psychology: Research and Practice* 38, no. 4 (2007), pp. 411–20; Anna Chur-Hansen and Deborah Zion, '"Let's Fix the Chemical Imbalance First, and Then We Can Work on the Problems Second": An Exploration of Ethical Implications of Prescribing an SSRI for "Depression"', *Monash Bioethics Review* 25, no. 1 (2006): 15–30; Brett J. Deacon and Grayson L. Baird, 'The Chemical Imbalance Explanation of Depression: Reducing Blame at What Cost?' *Journal of Social and Clinical Psychology* 28, no. 4 (2009): 415–35., in Harrington, p. 215.

46 Christopher Davey, 'The chemical imbalance theory of depression is dead – but that doesn't mean antidepressants don't work', *Guardian*, 2022.

47 J. Moncrieff, R. E. Cooper, T. Stockmann, et al., 'The serotonin theory of depression: a systematic umbrella review of the evidence', *Mol Psychiatry* (2022). doi.org/10.1038/s41380-022-01661-0

48 M. H. Teicher, C. Glod, J. O. Cole, 'Emergence of Intense Suicidal Preoccupation During Fluoxetine Treatment', *American Journal of Psychiatry*, 147, no. 2 (1990).

49 Rachel Schraer, Clare Hix & Lindsey Harris, 'Antidepressants: Two million taking them for five years or more', *BBC News*, 2023.

50 E. H. Turner, A. M. Matthews, E. Linardatos, R. A. Tell, R. Rosenthal, 'Selective publication of antidepressant trials and its influence on apparent efficacy', *N Engl J Med*. 358(3) (2008), pp. 252–60. doi: 10.1056/NEJMsa065779. PMID: 18199864.

51 'Antidepressants Can Cause "Chemical Castration"', *Mad in America*, 2023.

Notes

52 A. S. Bahrick, 'Persistence of sexual dysfunction side effects after discontinuation of antidepressant medications: Emerging evidence', *The Open Psychology Journal*, *1*, Article 42–50 (2008). doi. org/10.2174/1874350100801010042

53 Andrea Cipriani, MD, Prof Toshi A Furukawa, Georgia Salanti, Anna Chaimani, Lauren Z Atkinson, Yusuke Ogawa, et al., 'Comparative efficacy and acceptability of 21 antidepressant drugs for the acute treatment of adults with major depressive disorder: a systematic review and network meta-analysis', 391: 10128 (2018), pp. 1357–1366.

54 Álvaro Nuno Perez, Jose Suarez, Michel Le Bars, 'Sizing the Brain', Deloitte Insights, 2023.

55 *Evaluating the Brain Disease Model of Addiction*, (Eds) Nick Heather, Matt Field, Antony C. Moss and Sally Satel (London and New York: Routledge, 2022).

56 British Neuroscience Association, 2019.

57 H. Pashler, E. J. Wagenmakers , 'Editors' Introduction to the Special Section on Replicability in Psychological Science: A Crisis of Confidence?' *Perspect. Psychol. Sci.*7 (2012), pp. 528–530. doi: 10.1177/1745691612465253; Kelly, Robert E Jr and Matthew J Hoptman, 'Replicability in Brain Imaging', *Brain sciences* vol. 12,3 397 (2022) doi:10.3390/brainsci12030397.

58 G. Arrondo, N. F. Barrett, F. Güell, J. Bernacer, J. I. Murillo, 'Techne and Episteme: Challenges for a Fruitful Translation Between Neuroscience and Psychiatry', in: P. Gargiulo, H. Mesones Arroyo (eds) Psychiatry and Neuroscience Update. Springer, Cham (2019), p. 5.

59 M. Silver, G. Montana, T. E. Nichols, 'False positives in neuroimaging genetics using voxel-based morphometry data', *Neuroimage* 54 (2011), pp. 992–1000. doi:10.1016/j. neuroimage.2010.08.049.

60 Functional magnetic resonance imaging measures brain activity by detecting changes associated with blood flow that are linked to neuronal activation.

61 E. Sprooten, A. Rasgon, M. Goodman, A. Carlin, E. Leibu, W. H. Lee, et al., 'Addressing reverse inference in psychiatric neuroimaging: Meta-analyses of task-related brain activation in common mental disorders', *Hum Brain Mapp* (2016);0. doi:10.1002/ hbm.23486; R. A. Poldrack, C. I. Baker, J. Durnez, K. J. Gorgolewski, P. M. Matthews, M. R. Munafò, et al., 'Scanning the horizon:

towards transparent and reproducible neuroimaging research', *Nat Rev Neurosci* 18 (2017), pp. 115–26. doi:10.1038/nrn.2016.167; G. Arrondo, N. F. Barrett, F. Güell, J. Bernacer, J. I. Murillo, 'Techne and Episteme: Challenges for a Fruitful Translation Between Neuroscience and Psychiatry', in: P. Gargiulo, H. Mesones Arroyo (eds) 'Psychiatry and Neuroscience Update', *Springer*, Cham, (2019).

62 J. Paris, *Prescriptions for the mind: a critical view of contemporary psychiatry* (New York: Oxford University Press; 2008).

63 M. B. First, W. C. Drevets, C. Carter, D. P. Dickerstein, L. Kasoff, K. L. Kim, et al., 'Clinical Applications of Neuroimaging in Psychiatric Disorders', *Am J Psychiatry* 175 (2018), pp. 915–6. doi: 10.1176/appi.ajp.2018.1750701

64 Tom Insel, 'Understanding Mental Disorders as Circuit Disorders,' *National Institute of Mental Health*, 2010.

65 Ibid.

66 Alexis Madrigal, 'Scanning Dead Salmon in fMRI Machine Highlights Risk of Red Herrings', *Wired* (2009).

67 Kristen Martin, '"The Body Keeps the Score" offers uncertain science in the name of self-help. It's not alone', *The Washington Post* (2023).

68 Christian Jarrett, 'A Calm Look at the Most Hyped Concept in Neuroscience – Mirror Neurons', *Wired* (2013).

69 Kristen Martin, '"The Body Keeps the Score" offers uncertain science in the name of self-help. It's not alone', *The Washington Post* (2023).

70 C. Giebel, R. Corcoran, M. Goodall, et al., 'Do people living in disadvantaged circumstances receive different mental health treatments than those from less disadvantaged backgrounds?' *BMC Public Health* 20, 651 (2020). https://doi.org/10.1186/s12889-020-08820-4; T. von Soest, J. G. Bramness, W. Pedersen, L. Wichstrøm, 'The relationship between socio-economic status and antidepressant prescription: a longitudinal survey and register study of young adults', *Epidemiol Psychiatr Sci.* 21(1) (2012), pp. 87–95. doi: 10.1017/s2045796011000722. PMID: 22670416.

71 Denis Campbell, 'Strain on mental health care leaves 8m people without help, say NHS leaders', *Guardian* (29 August 2021).

72 'Modernising the Mental Health Act: Final report of the Independent Review of the Mental Health Act 1983', December 2018.

73 J. Das-Munshi, D. Bhugra & M. J. Crawford, 'Ethnic minority

inequalities in access to treatments for schizophrenia and schizoaffective disorders: findings from a nationally representative cross-sectional study', *BMC Med* **16**, 55 (2018). https://doi.org/10.1186/s12916-018-1035-5

74 Annabel Sowemimo, *Divided* (London: Profile, 2023) p. 205; Ashley Nellis, 'The Color of Justice: Racial and Ethnic Disparity in State Prisons', *The Sentencing Project* (October 2021).

75 James Lind Alliance. Parkinson's Top 10 Priorities [online] (2014).

76 L. Kennedy, H. Wilkinson, C. Henstridge, '"Buddy Pairs': a novel pilot scheme crafting knowledge exchange between biomedical dementia researchers and people affected by dementia – innovative practice', *Dementia* (2019).

3: The Myth of Personality Disorders: BPD

1 'Personality disorders and related traits', ICD-11 for Mortality and Morbidity Statistics: www.icd.who.int/dev11/l-m/en#!/http%3A%2F%2Fid.who.int%2Ficd%2Fentity%2F37291724

2 American Psychiatric Association (2013). *Diagnostic and statistical manual of mental disorders* (5th ed.). Washington, DC.

3 'Personality disorders and related traits', ICD-11 for Mortality and Morbidity Statistics: www.icd.who.int/dev11/l-m/en#!/http%3A%2F%2Fid.who.int%2Ficd%2Fentity%2F37291724.

4 I have opted for the term borderline personality disorder, as opposed to emotionally unstable personality disorder, which is the term used in the ICD, the DSM equivalent commissioned by the World Health Organisation, and the one more commonly used in the UK and Europe. The rationale for the ICD term was to simplify diagnosis and de-stigmatise the condition, but given the history of women being cast as hysterical, I don't see how this terminology of emotional instability really helps. I use the term borderline to draw attention to the concept's history, and because this remains the most commonly used term in psychiatry and society at large.

5 'DSM-IV and DSM-V Criteria for the Personality Disorders', American Psychiatric Association (2012).

6 Joel Paris, 'Suicidality in Borderline Personality Disorder', *Medicina (Kaunas, Lithuania)* vol. 55,6 223. 28 (2019), doi:10.3390/medicina55060223

7 O. Kernberg, *Borderline Conditions and Pathological Narcissism* (New York: Jason Aronson, 1975) in Stone, 2005, p. 9.

8 Stone, 2005, p. 9

9   Ibid.
10 Jack Drescher, M.D., 'What are Personality Disorders?' *American Psychiatric Association* (2022).
11 Stone, 2005, pp. 9–11,
12 R. E. Kendell, 'The distinction between personality disorder and mental illness', *British Journal of Psychiatry*. 180(2) (2002) pp. 110–115. doi:10.1192/bjp.180.2.110
13 Ibid.
14 M. A. Jimenez, 'Gender and Psychiatry: Psychiatric Conceptions of Mental Disorders in Women, 1960–1994', *Affilia*, 12(2). p. 163. doi:10.1177/088610999701200202
15 Lucas Fortaleza de Aquino Ferreira, Fábio Henrique Queiroz Pereira, Ana Maria Luna Neri Benevides, Matias Carvalho Aguiar Melo, 'Borderline personality disorder and sexual abuse: A systematic review', *Psychiatry Research*, Volume 262 (2018), pp. 70–77.
16 Ibid.
17 J. L. Herman, J. C. Perry, B. A. van der Kolk, 'Childhood trauma in borderline personality disorder', *Am J Psychiatry* 146(4) (1989), pp. 490–5. doi: 10.1176/ajp.146.4.490. PMID: 2929750.
18 Heather B. MacIntosh, Natacha Godbout, Nauveen Dubash, 'Borderline Personality Disorder: Disorder of Trauma or Personality, a Review of the Empirical Literature', *Canadian Psychology*, Vol. 56, No. 2 (2015) pp. 227–241.
19 Rose, 2019, p. 15.
20 Becker, 2000.
21 Devereux, Cecily. "Hysteria, Feminism, and Gender Revisited: The Case of the Second Wave." *ESC: English Studies in Canada*, vol. 40 no. 1, 2014, p. 19–45. *Project MUSE*, https://dx.doi.org/10.1353/esc.2014.0004.
22 Clare Shaw, 'Women at the Margins: A Critique of the Diagnosis of Borderline Personality Disorder', *Feminism & Psychology*, 15(4) (2005), pp. 483–490. https://doi.org/10.1177/0959-353505057620.
23 Showalter, 1985, pp. 3–4.
24 P. Chesler, *Women and Madness* (Garden City, NY: Doubleday, 1972).
25 Joel Paris, 'Suicidality in Borderline Personality Disorder', *Medicina (Kaunas, Lithuania)* vol. 55,6 223. 28 (2019), doi:10.3390/medicina55060223
26 X. Qian, M. L. Townsend, W. J. Tan, B. F. S. Grenyer, 'Sex differences

in borderline personality disorder: A scoping review', *PLoS ONE* 17(12) (2022). doi.org/10.1371/journal.pone.0279015

27 C. Rodriguez-Seijas, T. A. Morgan & M. Zimmerman, 'Is There a Bias in the Diagnosis of Borderline Personality Disorder Among Lesbian, Gay, and Bisexual Patients?' *Assessment*, 28(3) (2021), pp. 724–738. https://doi.org/10.1177/1073191120961833; M. L. Hatzenbuehler, J. E. Pachankis, 'Stigma and minority stress as social determinants of health among lesbian, gay, bisexual, and transgender youth: Research evidence and clinical implications', *Pediatric Clinics*, 63(6) (2016), pp. 985–997. https://doi.org/10.1016/j.pcl.2016.07.003; J. M. W. Hughto, S. L. Reisner, J. E. Pachankis, 'Transgender stigma and health: A critical review of stigma determinants, mechanisms, and interventions. *Social Science & Medicine*, 147 (2015), pp. 222–231. doi.org/10.1016/j.socscimed.2015.11.010

28 'Women's Mental Health: Into the Mainstream', *Department of Health* (2002).

29 Judith L. Herman, *Trauma and Recovery* (Basic Books/Hachette Book Group, 1992); Becker, D. *Through the Looking Glass: Women and BorderlinePpersonality Disorder* (Boulder, CO: Westview Press, 1997); C. Shaw, & G. I. Proctor, 'Women at the Margins: A Critique of the Diagnosis of Borderline Personality Disorder', *Feminism & Psychology*, 15(4) (2005), pp. 483–490. https://doi.org/10.1177/0959-353505057620

30 M. Cloitre, 'ICD-11 complex post-traumatic stress disorder: simplifying diagnosis in trauma populations', *The British Journal of Psychiatry*. 2020;216(3), pp.129–131. doi:10.1192/bjp.2020.43

31 Clare Shaw, 'Woman at the margins: me, Borderline Personality Disorder and Women at the Margins', *ANNUAL REVIEW OF CRITICAL PSYCHOLOGY* (2005), p. 131.

32 Shaw, 2005, p. 128.

33 E.g. O. D. Kothgassner, A. Goreis, K. Robinson, M. M. Huscsava, C. Schmahl, P. L. Plener, 'Efficacy of dialectical behavior therapy for adolescent self-harm and suicidal ideation: a systematic review and meta-analysis', *Psychological Medicine*, 51(7) (2021), pp. 1057–1067. doi:10.1017/S0033291721001355

34 E. Weight, and S. Kendal, 'Staff attitudes towards inpatients with borderline personality disorder', *Mental Health Practice*, Vol 17 issue 3 01 November 2013; E. Bodner, S. Cohen-Fridel, M. Mashiah, M. Segal, A. Grinshpoon, T. Fischel, et al. 'The attitudes of psychiatric

hospital staff toward hospitalization and treatment of patients with borderline personality disorder', *BMC Psychiatry* 15:2 (2015) doi:10.1186/s12888-014-0380-y; E. A. Kate, K. H. Saunders, S. Fortune, S. Farrell, 'Attitudes and knowledge of clinical staff regarding people who self-harm: a systematic review', *J Affect Disord* 139 (2012), pp. 205–16. doi:10.1016/j.jad.2011.08.024; Black DW, Pfohl B, Blum N, McCormick B, Allen J, North CS, et al. 'Attitudes toward borderline personality disorder: a survey of 706 mental health clinicians', *CNS Spectr* 16(3) (2011), pp. 67–74. doi:10.1017/S109285291200020X

35 L. Birmingham, 'The mental health of prisoners', *Advances in Psychiatric Treatment*, 9(3) (2003), pp. 191–199. doi:10.1192/apt.9.3.191

36 Courtney Conn et al. 'Borderline Personality Disorder Among Jail Inmates: How Common and How Distinct?' *Corrections compendium* vol. 35,4 (2010): pp. 6–13.

37 Estimated, based on: 'Rapid review into data on mental health inpatient settings: final report and recommendations', *Department of Health and Social Care* (March, 2024); https://www.nasmhpd.org/sites/default/files/2023-01/Trends-in-Psychiatric-Inpatient-Capacity_United-States%20_1970-2018_NASMHPD-2.pdf

38 R. Musgrove, M. Carr, N. Kapur, C. Chew-Graham, F. Mughal, D. Ashcroft and R. Webb, 'Suicide and other causes of death among working-age and older adults in the year after discharge from in-patient mental healthcare in England: Matched cohort study', *British Journal of Psychiatry*, 221:2, (2022), pp. 468–75; D. Osborn, G. Favarato, D. Lamb, T. Harper, S. Johnson, B. Lloyd-Evans and S. Weich, 'Readmission after discharge from acute mental healthcare among 231 988 people in England: Cohort study exploring predictors of readmission including availability of acute day units in local areas', *BJPsych Open*, 7(4):e136, (July 2021), in Mad World, Micha Frazer-Carroll, 2005, p. 153.

39 M. Morrow, 'Women, violence and mental illness: An evolving feminist critique', in: C. Patton, H. Loshny (eds) *Global Science/Women's Health* (New York: Cambria Press, 2008), pp. 147–162.

40 National Institute for Mental Health in England, 'Personality Disorder: No Longer a Diagnosis of Exclusion', *Department of Health* (2003).

41 Ibid.

42 National Institute for Health and Care Excellence, 'Antisocial Personality Disorder: Prevention and Management (Clinical

Guideline CG77)', *NICE* (2009); National Institute for Health and Care Excellence, 'Borderline Personality Disorder: Recognition and Management (Clinical Guideline CG78)', *NICE* (2009).

43 A. Tetley, M. Jinks, K. Howells, C. Duggan, M. McMurran, N. Huband, et al. 'A preliminary investigation of services for people with personality disorder in the East Midlands region of England', *Personal Ment Health* 6 (2012) pp. 33–44.

44 Micha Frazer-Carroll, *Mad World*, p. 166.

45 https://www.livingwellsystems.uk/trieste

46 Micha Frazer-Carroll, *Mad World*, p. 169.

47 Ibid.

48 E.g. in the UK: Rachel Hall, 'Mental health advance choice documents "would reduce sectioning"', *Guardian* (12 February 2024); 'Reform of The Mental Health Act in England and Wales', *Royal College of Psychiatrists* (2024).

49 Sophie K. Rosa, *Radical Intimacy* (London: Pluto Press, 2023) p. 32.

50 Ibid.

51 Micha Frazer-Carroll, *Mad World*, p. 107.

52 Merri Lisa Johnson, 'Neuroqueer Feminism: Turning with Tenderness toward Borderline Personality Disorder', *Signs: Journal of Women in Culture and Society*, 46:3 (2021), p. 644. doi:org/10.1086/712081

53 Johnson, 2021, p. 643.

54 Johnson, 2021, p. 645.

55 Christine Pungong, 'On The Realities of Being a Black Woman with Borderline Personality Disorder', *Fader* (March 2017).

4: The Blurred Lines of 'Female' Diagnoses: Postpartum Depression

1 Amalia Londoño Tobón, MD, 'What is Perinatal Depression?' *American Psychiatric Association* (2023).

2 Ibid.

3 Jonathan R. Scarff 'Postpartum Depression in Men', *Innovations in clinical neuroscience* vol. 16,5–6 (2019), pp. 11–14.

4 Saba Mughal, Yusra Azhar, Waquar Siddiqui, 'Postpartum Depression', *StatPearls*, Last Update: October 7, 2022.

5 E.g. 'Postnatal depression in dads: "I didn't know men could struggle too"', *BBC News* (19 November 2021). Ammar Kalia, '"I didn't even know men could get it": the hidden impact of male postnatal depression', *Guardian* (22 May 2023).

6 In the ICD-11, it is 6 weeks. See World Health Organisation (WHO)

(2019). International classification of diseases, eleventh revision (ICD-11). Available at: https://icd.who.int/

7   *American Psychiatric Association* (2013). 'Diagnostic and Statistical Manual of Mental Disorders' (5th ed.). Arlington, VA.; Saba Mughal; Yusra Azhar; Waquar Siddiqui, Postpartum Depression, *StatPearls*, Last Update: October 7, 2022.

8   D. N. Ugarriza, 'Postpartum depressed women's explanation of depression', *Journal of Nursing Scholarship*, 34 (2002), pp. 227–233. doi: 10.1111/j.1547-5069.2002.00227.x

9   D. L. Putnick, R. Sundaram, E. M. Bell, A. Ghassabian, R. B. Goldstein, S. L. Robinson, Y. Vafai, S. E. Gilman, E. Yeung, 'Trajectories of Maternal Postpartum Depressive Symptoms', *Pediatrics* 146(5) (2020). doi: 10.1542/peds.2020-0857.

10 R. Martinez, I. Johnston-Robledo, H. M. Ulsh & J. C. Chrisler, 'Singing "the baby blues": A content analysis of popular press articles about postpartum affective disturbances', *Women and Health*, 31 (2000), pp. 37–56; P. Nicolson, 'Understanding postnatal depression: A mother-centred approach', *Journal of Advanced Nursing*, 15 (1990), pp. 689–695. doi: 10.1111/1365-2648.ep8531591; S. Suda, E. Segi-Nishida, S. S. Newton & R. S. Duma, 'A postpartum model in rat: Behavioral and gene expression changes induces by ovarian steroid deprivation', *Biological Psychiatry*, 64 (2008), pp. 311–319. doi: 10.1016/j.biopsych.2008.03.029; Whiffen, 1992

11 J. Zonana & J. M. Gorman, 'The neurobiology of postpartum depression', *CNS Spectrums: The International Journal of Neuropsychiatric Medicine*, 10 (2005), pp. 792–799.

12 See Anne Fausto-Sterling's *Sexing the Body* (London: Basic Books, 2000) pp. 170–195 for a comprehensive history.

13 Fausto-Sterling, p. 170.

14 Fausto-Sterling, p. 28; p. 179; p. 193.

15 Marieke Bigg, *This Won't Hurt* (London: Hodder and Stoughton, 2023), pp. 93–94.

16 E.g. Elton Brás Camargo Júnior et al, 'Association between childhood trauma and postpartum depression among Brazilian puerperal women', *Rev. Latino-Am. Enfermagem*, 32 (2024); Y. Liu, L. Zhang, N. Guo et al. 'Postpartum depression and postpartum post-traumatic stress disorder: prevalence and associated factors', *BMC Psychiatry* 21, 487 (2021). doi.org/10.1186/s12888-021-03432-7

17 Katie Hazelgrove, Alessandra Biaggi, Freddie Waites, Montserrat Fuste, Sarah Osborne, Susan Conroy, Louise M. Howard, Mitul A.

Mehta, Maddalena Miele, Naghmeh Nikkheslat, Gertrude Seneviratne, Patricia A. Zunszain, Susan Pawlby, Carmine M. Pariante, Paola Dazzan, 'Risk factors for postpartum relapse in women at risk of postpartum psychosis: The role of psychosocial stress and the biological stress system', *Psychoneuroendocrinology*, Volume 128 (2021) doi.org/10.1016/j.psyneuen.2021.105218; M. Aas, C. Vecchio, A. Pauls, M. Mehta, S. Williams, K. Hazelgrove, A. Biaggi, S. Pawlby, S. Conroy, G. Seneviratne, V. Mondelli, C. M. Pariante, P. Dazzan, 'Biological stress response in women at risk of postpartum psychosis: The role of life events and inflammation', *Psychoneuroendocrinology* 113 (2020). doi: 10.1016/j.psyneuen.2019.104558. Epub 2019 Dec 19. PMID: 31923613.

18 O. S. Kowalczyk et al, 'Neurocognitive correlates of working memory and emotional processing in postpartum psychosis: an fMRI study', *Psychological Medicine* 51 (2021), pp. 1724–1732. doi.org/10.1017/ S0033291720000471

19 E.g. S. L. Mott, C. E. Schiller, J. G. Richards, M. W. O'Hara, S. Stuart, 'Depression and anxiety among postpartum and adoptive mothers', *Arch Womens Ment Health.* 14(4) (2011), pp. 335–43. doi: 10.1007/ s00737-011-0227-1; Yehuda Senecky, Hanoch Agassi, Dov Inbar, Netta Horesh, Gary Diamond, Yoav S. Bergman, Alan Apter, 'Post-adoption depression among adoptive mothers', *Journal of Affective Disorders*, Volume 115, Issues 1–2, 2009, pp. 62–68.

20 Y. Yu, H-F Liang, J. Chen, Z-B Li, Y-S Han, J-X Chen and J-C Li, 'Postpartum Depression: Current Status and Possible Identification Using Biomarkers', *Front. Psychiatry* 12:620371 (2021) doi: 10.3389/ fpsyt.2021.620371

21 Alkistis Skalkidou, Inger Sundström Poromaa, Stavros I. Iliadis, Anja C. Huizink, Charlotte Hellgren, Eva Freyhult, Erika Comasco, 'Stress-related genetic polymorphisms in association with peripartum depression symptoms and stress hormones: A longitudinal population-based study', *Psychoneuroendocrinology*, volume 103 (2019), pp. 296–305 doi.org/10.1016/j.psyneuen.2019.02.002; Y. B. Kofman, Z. E. Eng, D. Busse, S. Godkin, B. Campos, C. A. Sandman, D. Wing, I. S. Yim, 'Cortisol reactivity and depressive symptoms in pregnancy: The moderating role of perceived social support and neuroticism', *Biological Psychology* 147(SI) (2019).

22 E.g. Cheng, Ching-Yu, Yu-Hua Chou, Chia-Hao Chang, and Shwu-Ru Liou. 'Trends of Perinatal Stress, Anxiety, and Depression

and Their Prediction on Postpartum Depression', *International Journal of Environmental Research and Public Health* 18, no. 17: 9307 (2021). doi.org/10.3390/ijerph18179307; B. A. Baattaiah, M. D. Alharbi, N. M. Babteen, et al. 'The relationship between fatigue, sleep quality, resilience, and the risk of postpartum depression: an emphasis on maternal mental health', *BMC Psychol* 11, 10 (2023). doi. org/10.1186/s40359-023-01043-3; J. N. Felder, D. Roubinov, L. Zhang, et al. 'Endorsement of a single-item measure of sleep disturbance during pregnancy and risk for postpartum depression: a retrospective cohort study', *Arch Womens Ment Health* 26, 67–74 (2023). doi.org/10.1007/s00737-022-01287-9

23 L. Held, & A. Rutherford, 'Can't a mother sing the blues? Postpartum depression and the construction of motherhood in late 20th-century America', *History of Psychology*, 15 (2012), pp. 107–122. doi: 10.1037/a0026319, p. 119, in Alexander, 2013, p. 8.

24 Barnes, 2006; Beck, 2002, in Alexander, 2013, p. 15; Melissa Terry, 'Feminism, gender and women's experiences: Research approaches to address postnatal depression', *International Journal of Innovative Interdisciplinary Research*, V2 I3 (2014); Kherani, Imaan Zera, 'A feminist science commentary: a socially cognizant analysis of postpartum depression in the Western world', *University of Toronto Medical Journal*, Vol 98, Issue 2 (2021), p. 26.

25 Barnes, 2006; Elizabeth M. Alexander, 'Constructions of Motherhood and Fatherhood in Newspaper Articles on Maternal and Paternal Postpartum Depression', *Thesis, University of Saskatchewan* (2013).

26 C. Knudson-Martin & R. Silverstein, 'Suffering in silence: A qualitative meta-data analysis of postpartum depression', *Journal of Marital and Family Therapy* 35 (2009) 145–158; Alexander, 2013, p.15.

27 Alexander, 2013, p.16.

28 Barnes, 2006, p. 30; L. Held & A. Rutherford, 'Can't a mother sing the blues? Postpartum depression and the construction of motherhood in late 20th-century America. History of Psychology', 15 (2012), pp. 107–122 doi: 10.1037/a0026319, in Alexander, 2013, p. 15.

29 Alexander, 2013, p.16.

30 Ibid.

31 Alexander, 2013, pp. 13–17.

32 Ibid.

33 E.g. R. Canuso, 'Maternal depression: The "dual" diagnosis of mother and child', *Issues in Mental Health Nursing*, 29 (2008),

pp. 785–787. doi: 10.1080/01612840802129319; A. Stein, L.E. Malmberg, K. Sylva, J. Barnes, P. Leach & the FCCC team. 'The influence of maternal depression, caregiving, and socioeconomic status in the post-natal year on children's language development', *Child: Care, Health and Development*, 34 (2008), pp. 603–612. doi: 10.1111/j.1365-2214.2008.00837.x.

34 Held and Rutherford, 2012, p. 111, in Alexander, 2013, p. 15.

35 Knudson-Martin & Silverstein, 2009, in Alexander, 2013, p. 14.

36 R. Coates, S. Ayers & R. de Visser, 'Women's experiences of postnatal distress: a qualitative study', *BMC Pregnancy Childbirth* 14, 359 (2014). doi.org/10.1186/1471-2393-14-359; R. Coates, R. de Visser, S. Ayers, 'Not identifying with postnatal depression: a qualitative study of women's postnatal symptoms of distress and need for support', *J Psychosom Obstet Gynaecol* 36(3) (2015), pp. 114–21. doi: 10.3109/0167482X.2015.1059418.

37 Beck, 2002; Knudsen-Martin and Silverstein, 2009, in Alexander, 2013, p. 15.

38 Shuhei Terada, Kentaro Kinjo, Yoshiharu Fukuda, 'The relationship between postpartum depression and social support during the COVID-19 pandemic: A cross-sectional study', Volume 47, Issue 10 (2021) doi.org/10.1111/jog.14929, pp. 3524–3531; H. Cho, K. Lee, E. Choi, et al. 'Association between social support and postpartum depression', *Sci Rep* 12, 3128 (2022). doi.org/10.1038/s41598-022-07248-7; R. Bina, 'The impact of cultural factors upon postpartum depression: A literature review', *Health Care for Women International* 29 (2008), pp. 568–592. doi: 10.1080/07399330802089149; S. M. Haga, A. Lynne, K. Slinning & P. Kraft, 'A qualitative study of depressive symptoms and well-being among first-time mothers', *Scandinavian Journal of Caring Sciences*, 26 (2012), pp. 458–466. doi: 10.1111/j.1471-6712.2011.00950.x; R. Negron, A. Martin, M. Almog, A. Balbierz & E. Howell, 'Social support during the postpartum period: Mothers' views on needs, expectations, and mobilization of support', *Maternal & Child Health Journal*, 17 (2013), pp. 616–623. doi: 10.1007/s10995-012-1037-4; B. Posmontier & J. A. Horowitz, 'Postpartum practices and depression prevalences: Technocentric and ethnokinship cultural perspectives', *Journal of Transcultural Nursing*, 15 (2004), pp. 34–43. doi: 10.1177/1043659603260032; D. Lasek, 'Mother-daughter attachment, social support, relationship with husband, and socioeconomic status as predictors of postpartum' (2000); Logsdon,

M., J. C. Birkimer & W. Usui, 'The link of social support and postpartum depressive symptoms in African-American women with low incomes', *American Journal of Maternal Child Nursing*, 25(5) (2000), pp. 262–266; M. Marks & K. Siddle, 'A randomized controlled trial to assess the effect of specialized midwifery care' (2000). Paper presented at the Marce Society Conference, Manchester, England; S. Misri, X. Kostaras, D. Fox & D. Kostaras, 'The impact of partner support in the treatment of postpartum depression', *Canadian Journal of Psychiatry – Revue Canadienne de Psychiatrie*, 45(6) (2000), pp. 554–558; Z. Stowe & C. Nemeroff, 'Women at risk for postpartum-onset major depression', *American Journal of Obstetrics & Gynecology*, 173(2) (1995), pp. 639–645; W. Wolman, B. Chalmers, G. Hofmeyr & V. Nikodem, 'Postpartum depression and companionship in the clinical birth environment: A randomized, controlled study', *American Journal of Obstetrics & Gynecol- ogy*, 168(5) (1993), pp. 1388–1393; B. Cheng, N. Roberts, Y. Zhou, et al. 'Social support mediates the influence of cerebellum functional connectivity strength on postpartum depression and postpartum depression with anxiety', *Transl Psychiatry* 12, 54 (2022). doi.org/10.1038/s41398-022-01781-9

39 S. Kim, D. J. Kim, M. S. Lee, H. Lee, 'Association of Social Support and Postpartum Depression According to the Time After Childbirth in South Korea', *Psychiatry Investig* 20(8) (2023), pp. 750–757. doi: 10.30773/pi.2023.0042; J. Żyrek, M. Klimek, A. Apanasewicz, et al. 'Social support during pregnancy and the risk of postpartum depression in Polish women: A prospective study', *Sci Rep* 14, 6906 (2024). doi.org/10.1038/s41598-024-57477-1; H. Cho, K. Lee, E. Choi et al. 'Association between social support and postpartum depression', *Sci Rep* 12, 3128 (2022). doi.org/10.1038/s41598-022-07248-7; Mandu Stephen Ekpenyong, Munshitha Munshitha, 'The impact of social support on postpartum depression in Asia: A systematic literature review', *Mental Health & Prevention*, volume 30 (2023).

40 L. E. Ross, L. Steele, C. Goldfinger, C. Strike, 'Perinatal depressive symptomatology among lesbian and bisexual women', *Archives of Women's Mental Health*, 10 (2007), pp. 53–59.

41 M. E. Silverman, H. Loudon, 'Antenatal reports of pre-pregnancy abuse is associated with symptoms of depression in the postpartum period', *Archives of Women's Mental Health*, 13 (2010), pp. 411–415.

42 J. Milgrom, A. W. Gemmill, J. L. Bilszta, B. Hayes B, B. Barnett B, J.

Notes

Brooks et al. 'Antenatal risk factors for postnatal depression: A large prospective study', *Journal of Affective* Disorders, 108 (2008), pp. 147–157; L. E. Ross, 'Perinatal mental health in lesbian mothers: a review of potential risk and protective factors', *Women Health*, 41(3) (2005), pp. 113–28. doi: 10.1300/J013v41n03_07; L. S. Steele, L. E. Ross, R. Epstein, C. Strike & C. Goldfinger, 'Correlates of mental health service use among lesbian, gay, and bisexual mothers and prospective mothers', *Women & Health*, 47 (2008), pp. 95–112.

43 P. Boyce, A. Hickey, 'Psychosocial risk factors to major depression after childbirth', *Social Psychiatry and Psychiatric Epidemiology*, 40 (2005), pp. 605–612.

44 Ibid.

45 E.g. M. E. Silverman, H. Loudon, 'Antenatal reports of pre-pregnancy abuse is associated with symptoms of depression in the postpartum period', *Archives of Women's Mental Health*, 13 (2010), pp. 411–415.

46 Elaine M. Maccio, PhD and Jaimee A. Pangburn, MSW, 'The Case for Investigating Postpartum Depression in Lesbians and Bisexual Women', *Women's Health Issues*, VOLUME 21, ISSUE 3 (2011), p. 187–190. doi.org/10.1016/j.whi.2011.02.007

47 L. Adler, I. Yehoshua, M. Mizrahi Reuveni, 'Postpartum Depression Among Gay Fathers With Children Born Through Surrogacy: A Cross-sectional Study', *J Psychiatr Pract.* 29(1) (2023), pp. 3–10. doi: 10.1097/PRA.0000000000000684; L. Huller Harari, U. Blasbalg, S. Arnon, J. Ben-Sheetrit, P. Toren P, 'Risk factors for postpartum depression among sexual minority and heterosexual parents', *Australasian Psychiatry.* 30(6) (2022), pp. 718–721. doi:10.1177/10398562221133990

48 Smitha Mundasad, 'Black women four times more likely to die in childbirth', BBC News (11 November 2021).

49 'Issue Brief: Black Maternal Mental Health', *The Policy Center for Maternal Mental Health* (December 11 2023).

50 Tobi Thomas, 'Black mothers twice as likely as white mothers to be hospitalised with perinatal mental illness', *Guardian* (6 May 2024).

51 Aynur Kızılırmak, Pelin Calpbinici, Gülin Tabakan & Bahtışen Kartal, 'Correlation between postpartum depression and spousal support and factors affecting postpartum depression', *Health Care for Women International*, 42:12 (2021), pp. 1325–1339, DOI: 10.1080/07399332.2020.1764562; M. Grube, 'Inpatient treatment of women with postpartum psychiatric disorders – the role of male

partners', *Archives of Women's Mental Health*, 8 (2005), pp. 163–170. doi: 10.1007/s00737-005-0087-7; T. Uçar, Z. Bal, N. Gökbulut, E. C. Kantar, E. Güney, 'The relationship between social support and spousal support perceived by women in the postpartum period and readiness for discharge', *Genel Tıp Dergisi.* 32(2) (2022), pp. 190–197.

52 Alexander, 2013, p. 9.

53 E.g. J. H. Goodman, 'Paternal postpartum depression, its relationship to maternal postpartum depression, and implication for family health', *Journal of Advanced Nursing*, 45 (2004), pp. 26–35. doi: 10.1046/j.1365-2648.2003.02857.x; R. T. Pinheiro, P. V. S. Magalhaes, B. L. Horta, K. A. T. Pinheiro, R. A. da Silva & R. H. Pinto, 'Is paternal postpartum depression associated with maternal postpartum depression: Population-based study in Brazil', *Acta Psychiatrica Scandinavica*, 113 (2006), pp. 230–232. doi: 10.1111/j.1600-0447.2005.00708.x; C. Ballard & R. Davies, 'Postnatal depression in fathers', *International Review of Psychiatry*, 8 (1996), pp. 65–71; N. Letourneau, L. Duffet-Leger, C-L Dennis, M. Stewart & P. D. Tryphonopoulos, 'Identifying the support needs of fathers affected by postpartum depression: A pilot study', *Journal of Psychiatric and Mental Health Nursing*, 18 (2011), pp. 41–47. doi: 10.1111/j.1365-2850.2010.01627.x: 10.1097/CHI.ob013e31816429c2; S. L. Roberts, J. A. Bushnell, S. C. Collings & G. L. Purdie, 'Psychological health of men with partners who have post-partum depression', *The Australian and New Zealand Journal of Psychiatry*, 40 (2006), pp. 704–711. doi: 10.1080/j.1440-1614.2006.01871.x, in Alexander, 2013. S. P. Thomas, 'Perinatal depression in men', *Issues in Mental Health Nursing*, 31 (2010), p. 621. doi: 10.3109/01612840.2010.509988

54 V. Escriba-Aguir & L. Artazcoz, 'Gender differences in postpartum depression: A longitudinal cohort study', *Journal of Epidemiology & Community Health*, 65 (2011), pp. 320–326. doi: 10.1136/jech.2008.085894

55 E.g. Ozra Barooj-Kiakalaee, Seyed-Hamzeh Hosseini, Reza-Ali Mohammadpour-Tahmtan, Monirolsadate Hosseini-Tabaghdehi, Shayesteh Jahanfar, Zahra Esmaeili-Douki, Zohreh Shahhosseini, 'Paternal postpartum depression's relationship to maternal pre and postpartum depression, and father-mother dyads marital satisfaction: A structural equation model analysis of a longitudinal study', *Journal of Affective Disorders*, volume 297 (2022), pp. 375–380, doi.org/10.1016/j.jad.2021.10.110; Pérez C F, Brahm M P. 'Paternal postpartum depression: Why is it also important?' *Revista Chilena*

de Pediatria. 88(5) (2017), pp. 582–585. DOI: 10.4067/s0370-41062017000500002; Goodman, 2004; Letourneau, N., Duffet-Leger, L., Dennis, C.-L., Stewart, M. & Tryphonopoulos, P.D. 'Identifying the support needs of fathers affected by postpartum depression: A pilot study', *Journal of Psychiatric and Mental Health Nursing*, 18 (2011), pp. 41–47. doi: 10.1111/j.1365-2850.2010.01627.x

56 Ibid; F. Thiel, M-M Pittelkow, H-U Wittchen and S. Garthus-Niegel, 'The Relationship Between Paternal and Maternal Depression During the Perinatal Period: A Systematic Review and Meta-Analysis', *Front. Psychiatry* 11:563287 (2020). doi: 10.3389/fpsyt.2020.563287

57 Dan Wang, Yi-Lu Li, Dan Qiu, Shui-Yuan Xiao, 'Factors Influencing Paternal Postpartum Depression: A Systematic Review and Meta-Analysis', *Journal of Affective Disorders*, volume 293 (2021), pp. 51–63 doi.org/10.1016/j.jad.2021.05.088; Marina Schumacher, Carlos Zubaran, Gillian White, 'Bringing birth-related paternal depression to the fore', *Women and Birth*, Volume 21, Issue 2 (2008), pp. 65–70, doi.org/10.1016/j.wombi.2008.03.008; Francisca Pérez C., Paulina Brahm, Soledad Riquelme, Claudia Rivera, Karina Jaramillo, Andreas Eickhorst, 'Paternal post-partum depression: How has it been assessed? A literature review', *Mental Health & Prevention*,Volume 7 (2017), pp. 28–36.

58 Michael B. Wells, Olov Aronson, 'Paternal postnatal depression and received midwife, child health nurse, and maternal support: A cross-sectional analysis of primiparous and multiparous fathers', *Journal of Affective Disorders*, Volume 280, Part A (2021), pp. 127–135, doi.org/10.1016/j.jad.2020.11.018; S. Melrose, 'Paternal postpartum depression: How can nurses begin to help?' *Contemporary Nurse*, 34 (2010), pp. 199–210; S. A. Madsen, 'Men's mental health: Fatherhood and psychotherapy', *The Journal of Men's Studies*, 17 (2009), pp. 15–30. doi: 10.3149/jms.1701.15.

59 Darby E. Saxbe, Robin S. Edelstein, Hannah M. Lyden, Britney M. Wardecker, William J. Chopik, Amy C. Moors, 'Fathers' decline in testosterone and synchrony with partner testosterone during pregnancy predicts greater postpartum relationship investment', *Hormones and Behavior*, Volume 90 (201), pp. 39–47, doi.org/10.1016/j.yhbeh.2016.07.005; Sandra J. Berg, Katherine E. Wynne-Edwards, 'Changes in Testosterone, Cortisol, and Estradiol Levels in Men Becoming Fathers', *Mayo Clinic Proceedings*, Volume 76, Issue 6 (2001), pp. 582–592, doi.org/10.4065/76.6.582.

60 Ibid.
61 F. A. Zarrouf, S. Artz, J. Griffith et al. 'Testosterone and depression: systematic review and meta-analysis', *J Psychiatr Pract.* 15(4) (2009), pp. 289–305; P. Kim, J. E. Swain, 'Sad dads: paternal postpartum depression', *Psychiatry (Edgmont)* 4(2) (2007), pp. 35–47.
62 Emily E. Cameron, Dana Hunter, Ivan D. Sedov, Lianne M. Tomfohr-Madsen, 'What do dads want? Treatment preferences for paternal postpartum depression', *Journal of Affective Disorders*, Volume 215 (2017), pp. 62–70, doi.org/10.1016/j.jad.2017.03.031.
63 B. M. Kuehn, 'Postpartum Depression Screening Needs More Consistency', *JAMA.* 323(24) (2020), p. 2454. doi:10.1001/jama.2020.9737
64 Dawn Edge, 'Ethnicity, psychosocial risk, and perinatal depression – a comparative study among inner-city women in the United Kingdom', *Journal of Psychosomatic Research*, Volume 63, Issue 3 (2007), pp. 291–295, doi.org/10.1016/j.jpsychores.2007.02.013; 'Mental health care during pregnancy and afterwards: women from some ethnic minority backgrounds face barriers to access', National Institute for Health and Care Research (April 2021); Floyd James, Kortney, Betsy E. Smith, Millicent N. Robinson, Courtney S. Thomas Tobin, Kelby F. Bulles, and Jennifer L. Barkin. 'Factors Associated with Postpartum Maternal Functioning in Black Women: A Secondary Analysis,' *Journal of Clinical Medicine* 12, no. 2 (2023), p. 647. doi.org/10.3390/jcm12020647; S. Liu, X. Ding, A. Belouali, H. Bai, K. Raja, H. Kharrazi, 'Assessing the Racial and Socioeconomic Disparities in Postpartum Depression Using Population-Level Hospital Discharge Data: Longitudinal Retrospective Study', *JMIR Pediatr Parent* 5(4) (2022).
65 'Saving Lives, Improving Mothers' Care Lay Summary 2021', *NPEU* (2021).
66 E. Kennedy, K. Munyan, 'Sensitivity and reliability of screening measures for paternal postpartum depression: an integrative review', *J Perinatol* 41 (2021), pp. 2713–2721. doi.org/10.1038/s41372-021-01265-6

5: Psychiatric Impossibilities: Psychopathy

1 In Gabor Maté, *The Myth of Normal* (London: Vermillion, 2022). p. 307.
2 K. A. Kiehl, M. B. Hoffman, 'The criminal psychopath: history, neuroscience, treatment, and economics', *Jurimetrics.* 51 (2011),

pp. 355–397; James Blair, Derek Mitchell and Karina Blair, *The Psychopath: Emotion and the Brain* (Malden: Blackwell, 2005).

3   This is based on estimates that 1 per cent of all noninstitutionalised men age 18 and over are psychopaths, according to the Hare psychopath test. This means 1,150,000 adult males in the US. Of the 6,720,000 men in prison, 16 per cent, or 1,075,000 are said to be psychopaths. This leads to the figure of 93 per cent for the adult male psychopath population in jail. All these results are based on criteria and scales that have been challenged, and estimates based on little actual research. See, Kiehl KA, Hoffman MB. 'The criminal psychopath: history, neuroscience, treatment, and economics', *Jurimetrics.* 51 (2011), pp. 355–397.

4   Nicholas D. Thomson, *Understanding Psychopathy: The Biopsychosocial Perspective* (London: Routledge, 2019), p. 3.

5   Tonia L.G. Nicholls, Ivy Goossens, Candice L. Dodgers, David J. Cooke, 'Women and Girls with Psychopathic Characteristics', pp. 465–505, in A. Felthous & H. Sass (Eds.). *The Wiley international handbook on psychopathic disorders and the law* (2nd ed.) (London: Wiley-Blackwell, 2020).

6   Thomson, 2019, p. 3.

7   K. A. Kiehl, M. B. Hoffman, 'The criminal psychopath: history, neuroscience, treatment, and economics', *Jurimetrics.* 51 (2011), pp. 355–397.

8   Ibid; K. A. Kiehl, *The Psychopath Whisperer: The Science of Those Without Conscience* (Oneworld Publications, 2013).

9   A. Sanz-García, C. Gesteira, J. Sanz, M. P. García-Vera, 'Prevalence of Psychopathy in the General Adult Population: A Systematic Review and Meta-Analysis', *Front Psychol.* 12 (2021). doi: 10.3389/fpsyg.2021.661044.

10 Daniel Boduszek, Agata Debowska, 'Critical evaluation of psychopathy measurement (PCL-R and SRP-III/SF) and recommendations for future research', *Journal of Criminal Justice*, Volume 44 (2016), pp. 1–12, ISSN 0047-2352, doi.org/10.1016/j.jcrimjus.2015.11.004.

11 D. J. Cooke & C. Michie, 'Psychopathy across cultures: North America and Scotland compared', *Journal of Abnormal Psychology*, 108(1) (1999), pp. 58–68. doi.org/10.1037/0021-843X.108.1.58

12 S. V. Shariat, S. M. Assadi, M. Noroozian, M. Pakravannejad, O. Yahyazadeh, S. Aghayan, C. Michie, D. Cooke, 'Psychopathy in Iran:

a cross-cultural study', *J Pers Disord.* 24(5) (2010), pp. 676–91. doi: 10.1521/pedi.2010.24.5.676. PMID: 20958175.

13 E. Forouzan, 'Psychopathy among women: Conceptualisation and assessment problems', *Third Annual International Association of Forensic Mental Health Services (IAFMHS) Conference, Miami, FL.* (2003).

14 Ibid.

15 E. M. Cale & S. O. Lilienfeld, 'Sex differences in psychopathy and antisocial personality disorder – A review and integration', *Clinical Psychology Review*, 22(8) (2002), pp. 1179–1207. doi:10.1016/s0272-7358(01)00125-8; V. de Vogel & M. Lancel, 'Gender differences in the assessment and manifestation of psychopathy: results from a multicenter study in forensic psychiatric patients', *International Journal of Forensic Mental Health*, 15(1) (2016), pp. 97–110. doi:10.1080 /14999013.2016.1138173; E. Forouzan & D. J. Cooke, 'Figuring out la femme fatale: Conceptual and assessment issues concerning psychopathy in females', *Behavioral Sciences and the Law*, 23(6) (2005), pp. 765–778. doi:10.1002/bsl.669; C. Logan, 'Psychopathy in Women: Conceptual Issues, Clinical Presentation and Management', *Neuropsychiatrie*, 23 (2009), pp. 25–33; E. Verona & J. Vitale, 'Psychopathy in women. In C. J. Patrick (Ed.), *Handbook of psychopathy* (New York: Guilford Press, 2006), pp. 415–436; Steven M. Gillespie, Carlo Garofalo, Luna C.M. Centifanti, 'Variants of psychopathy in male and female civil psychiatric patients: Latent profile analyses of the MacArthur violence risk dataset', *Journal of Criminal Justice*, Volume 72 (2021), doi.org/10.1016/j. jcrimjus.2020.101748.

16 C. Logan & G. Weizmann-Henelius, 'Psychopathy in women: Presentation, assessment and management' in H. Ha'kka'nen-Nyholm and J. O. Nyholm (Eds.) *Psychopathy and the law* (Chichester: John Wiley and Sons, 2012), pp. 99–126; M. Grann, 'The PCL–R and gender', *European Journal of Psychological Assessment*, 16(3), (2000), pp. 147–149; Forouzan & Cooke, 2005; M. K. Kreis & D. J. Cooke, 'Capturing the psychopathic female: A prototypicality analysis of the Comprehensive Assessment of Psychopathic Personality (CAPP) across gender', *Behavioral Sciences & the Law*, 29(5) (2011), pp. 634–648; Logan & Weizmann-Henelius, 2012.

17 K. A. Kiehl, M. B. Hoffman, 2011, pp. 355–397.

18 SENT'G PROJECT, REPORT OF THE SENTENCING PROJECT

TO THE UNITED NATIONS SPECIAL RAPPORTEUR ON
CONTEMPORARY FORMS OF RACISM, RACIAL
DISCRIMINATION, XENOPHOBIA, AND RELATED
INTOLERANCE 1 (March 2018) www.sentencingproject.org/
wp-content/uploads/2018/04/UN-Report-onRacial-Disparities.pdf
[https://perma.cc/SF8B-W4LN.

19 Gabriella Argueta-Cevallos, 'A prosecutor with a smoking gun:
examining the weaponization of race, psychopathy, and ASPD
labels in capital cases', *Columbia Human Rights Law Review* (2022),
p. 647.

20 A. R. Fox, T. H. Kvaran, R. G. Fontaine, 'Psychopathy and
Culpability: How Responsible Is the Psychopath for Criminal
Wrongdoing?' *Law & Social Inquiry* 38(1) (2013), pp. 1–26. doi:10.1111/
j.1747-4469.2012.01294.x; Lisa G. Aspinwall et al. 'The Double-Edged
Sword: Does Biomechanism Increase or Decrease Judges'
Sentencing of Psychopaths?' *Science* 337 (2012), pp. 846–849.

21 'Working with People in the Criminal Justice System Showing
Personality Disorders', *NHS* (2020). www.assets.publishing.service.
gov.uk/government/uploads/system/uploads/attachment_data/
file/1035881/6.5151_HMPPS_Working_with_Offenders_with_
Personality_Disorder_accessible_version_.pdf

22 PCL, R. D. Hare, 'A research scale for the assessment of
psychopathy in criminal populations', *Personality and Individual
Differences*, *1*(2) (1980), pp. 111–119; PCL-R, R. D. Hare, *The Hare
Psychopathy Checklist-Revised: Manual* (Toronto: Multi-Health
Systems, Incorporated, 1991); PCL:SV, Hart, S., Cox, D. & Hare, R.
Manual for the Psychopathy Checklist: Screening version (PCL: SV)
(Toronto: Multi-Health Systems, 1995).

23 D. J. Cooke & C. Logan, 'Capturing psychopathic personality:
Penetrating the mask of sanity through clinical interview' in C. J.
Patrick (Ed.) *Handbook of Psychopathy* (2nd ed.) (New York, NY:
The Guilford Press, 2018), pp. 189–210.

24 When using the CAPP test, on the other hand, the researchers
identified both patients as psychopathic. See Mette K. F. Kreis &
David J. Cooke, 'The Manifestation of Psychopathic Traits in
Women: An Exploration Using Case Examples', *International
Journal of Forensic Mental Health*, 11:4, (2012), pp. 267–279.

25 E. Forouzan, 'Psychopathy among women: Conceptualisation and
assessment problems', *Third Annual International Association of*

Forensic Mental Health Services (IAFMHS) Conference, Miami, FL. (2003).

26 B. T. Kerridge, R. P. Pickering, T. D. Saha, W. J. Ruan, S. P. Chou, H. Zhang, J. Jung, D. S. Hasin, 'Prevalence, sociodemographic correlates and DSM-5 substance use disorders and other psychiatric disorders among sexual minorities in the United States', *Drug Alcohol Depend.* 170 (2017), pp. 82–92. doi 10.1016/j. drugalcdep.2016.10.038; Sandfort TG, de Graaf R, Ten Have M, Ransome Y, Schnabel P. 'Same-sex sexuality and psychiatric disorders in the second Netherlands Mental Health Survey and Incidence Study (NEMESIS-2)', *LGBT Health.* 1(4) (2014), pp. 292–301. doi: 10.1089/lgbt.2014.0031.

27 K. A. Fisher, T. J. Torrico, M. Hany, 'Antisocial Personality Disorder' in: *Treasure Island* (FL: StatPearls Publishing, 2024).

28 D. J. Cooke, S. D. Hart, C. Logan & C. Michie, 'Explicating the construct of psychopathy: Development and validation of a conceptual model, the Comprehensive Assessment of Psychopathic Person- ality (CAPP)', *International Journal of Forensic Mental Health*, 11(4) (2012), pp. 242–252.

29 For studies showing how the CAPP diagnoses psychopathy across gender, see M. K. Kreis & D. J. Cooke, 'Capturing the psychopathic female: A prototypicality analysis of the Comprehensive Assessment of Psychopathic Personality (CAPP) across gender', *Behavioral Sciences & the Law*, 29(5) (2011), pp. 634–648; M. K. Kreis, D. J. Cooke, C. Michie, H. A. Hoff & C. Logan, 'The Comprehensive Assessment of Psychopathic Personality (CAPP): Content validation using prototypical analysis', *Journal of Personality Disorders*, 26(3) (2012), pp. 402–413; L. Pedersen, C. Kunz, K. Rasmussen & P. Elsass, 'Psychopathy as a risk factor for violent recidivism: Investigating the Psychopathy Checklist Screening Version (PCL: SV) and the Comprehensive Assessment of Psychopathic Personality (CAPP) in a forensic psychiatric setting', *International Journal of Forensic Mental Health*, 9(4) (2010), pp. 308–315.

30 Robert D. Hare and Craig S. Neumann, 'Psychopathy as a Clinical and Empirical Construct', *Annual Review of Clinical Psychology* 4:1 (2008), pp. 217–246; Patrick CJ, Drislane LE. 'Triarchic Model of Psychopathy: Origins, Operationalizations, and Observed Linkages with Personality and General Psychopathology', *J Pers.* 83(6) (2015), pp. 627–43. doi: 10.1111/jopy.12119; J. Coid, M. Yang, S. Ullrich, A.

Roberts, R. D. Hare, 'Prevalence and correlates of psychopathic traits in the household population of Great Britain', *International Journal of law and Psychiatry.* 32(2) (2009), pp. 65–73. DOI: 10.1016/j.ijlp.2009.01.002. PMID: 19243821; A. Sanz-García, C. Gesteira, J. Sanz, M. P. García-Vera, 'Prevalence of Psychopathy in the General Adult Population: A Systematic Review and Meta-Analysis', *Front Psychol.* 12:661044 (2021) doi: 10.3389/fpsyg.2021.661044.

31 Jeremy Coid, Min Yang, Simone Ullrich, Amanda Roberts, Robert D. Hare, 'Prevalence and correlates of psychopathic traits in the household population of Great Britain', *International Journal of Law and Psychiatry*, Volume 32, Issue 2 (2009), pp. 65–73, doi. org/10.1016/j.ijlp.2009.01.002.

32 M. K. Kreis & D. J. Cooke, 'Capturing the psychopathic female: A prototypicality analysis of the Comprehensive Assessment of Psychopathic Personality (CAPP) across gender', *Behavioral Sciences & the Law*, 29(5) (2011), p. 645.

33 Sprague, Jenessa et al. 'Borderline personality disorder as a female phenotypic expression of psychopathy?' *Personality disorders* vol. 3,2 (2012), pp. 127–39. doi:10.1037/a0024134

34 Synergi, 'The impact of racism on mental health, briefing paper' (2018).

35 A. McGilloway, R. E. Hall, T. Lee et al. 'A systematic review of personality disorder, race and ethnicity: prevalence, aetiology and treatment', *BMC Psychiatry* 10, 33 (2010). doi. org/10.1186/1471-244X-10-33

36 A. Hossain, M. Malkov, T. Lee, K. Bhui, 'Ethnic variation in personality disorder: evaluation of 6 years of hospital admissions', *BJPsych Bull.* 42(4) (2018), pp. 157–161. doi: 10.1192/bjb.2018.31.

37 Randall T. Salekin, 'Psychopathy and therapeutic pessimism Clinical lore or clinical reality?' *Clinical Forensic Psychology and Law*, 1st ed (London: Routledge, 2007).

38 M. Caldwell, J. Skeem, R. Salekin & G. Van Rybroek, 'Treatment Response of Adolescent Offenders With Psychopathy Features: A 2-Year Follow-Up', *Criminal Justice and Behavior*, 33(5) (2006), pp. 571–596. doi.org/10.1177/0093854806288176; Christopher J. Patrick (ed), *Handbook of Psychopathy* (New York and London: The Guilford Press, 2018); S. A. De Brito, A. E. Forth, A. R. Baskin-Sommers et al. 'Psychopathy', *Nat Rev Dis Primers* 7, 49 (2021). doi. org/10.1038/s41572-021-00282-1

39 Jenny Tew and Alice Bennett, 'The Chromis programme:

Exploratory research using multiple case studies', Psychology Services, Her Majesty's Prison and Probation Service and Louise Dixon, School of Psychology, Victoria University of Wellington Ministry of Justice Analytical Series (2020).

40 J. Tew, L. Dixon, L. Harkins & A. Bennett, 'Investigating changes in anger and aggression in offenders with high levels of psychopathic traits attending the Chromis violence reduction programme', *Criminal Behaviour and Mental Health.* 22. (2012), pp.191–201.

41 James Fallon, *The Psychopath Inside* (London: Penguin, 2014).

42 T. L. Nicholls, K. R. Cruise, D. Greig & H. Hinz, 'Female offenders', In B. L. Cutler & P. A. Zapf (Eds.), *APA Handbook of Forensic Psychology* (Vol. 2) (Washington, DC, USA: American Psychological Association, 2015) pp. 79–123.

43 E. L. Robertson, J. V. Ray, P. J. Frick et al. 'The bidirectional effects of antisocial behaviour, anxiety, and trauma exposure: Implications for our understanding of the development of callous-unemotional traits', *Journal of Psychopathology and Clinical Science* (2023). doi: 10.1037/abn0000815. PMID: 36951750.

44 E. Forouzan & T. L. Nicholls, 'Childhood and adolescent characteristics of women with high versus low psychopathy scores: Examining developmental precursors to the malignant personality disorder', *Journal of Criminal Justice, 43*(4) (2015), pp. 307–320.

45 Jerome Groopman, 'The Troubled History of Psychiatry', *The New Yorker* (20 May 2019).

46 Rose, 2019, p. 187

47 Nikolas Rose, *Our Psychiatric Future* (London: Polity Press, 2019) p. 92, 182.

48 An interesting example on psychopathic traits in police officers: D. M. Falkenbach, J. Balash, M. Tsoukalas, S. Stern & S. O. Lilienfeld, 'From theoretical to empirical: Considering reflections of psychopathy across the thin blue line', *Personality Disorders: Theory, Research, and Treatment, 9*(5) (2018), pp. 420–428. doi.org/10.1037/per0000270

49 R. T. Salekin, C. Worley, R. D. Grimes, 'Treatment of psychopathy: a review and brief introduction to the mental model approach for psychopathy', *Behav Sci Law.* 28(2) (2010), pp. 235–66. doi: 10.1002/bsl.928.

50 Megha Mohan, 'What it's like living as a female psychopath', *BBC Online* (14 November 2022).

6: The Biological Dream

1   J. Read, 'Does "Schizophrenia" Exist? Reliability and Validity', in J. Read & J. Dillon (Eds.), *Models of Madness: Psychological, Social and Biological Approaches to Psychosis* (2nd ed.) (London: Routledge, 2013), pp. 47–61

2   McNally, *A Critical History of Schizophrenia* (London: Macmillan, 2016).

3   Gottesman and Shields, 1972, in McNally, *A Critical History of Schizophrenia*, 2016.

4   Symptoms are the behaviours or physical signs that are believed to indicate a disease. A psychiatric disorder is a set of related behavioural, emotional, or cognitive symptoms that are not readily controlled by the individual and are deemed 'clinically significant' in that they impair someone's ability to work, maintain relationships and participate in society. A syndrome is similarly a group of symptoms, but unlike a disorder, does to have a clear cause. A spectrum approach treats a disorder more like a syndrome, consisting of subgroups, which vary but are considered to be linked. The spectrum may also reflect varying degrees of severity. Psychogenic disorders are classified as 'conversion disorders', which are characterised by neurological symptoms with no identified underlying disease causing them. Examples are loss of strength in a limb, convulsions, or a loss of sensation. This classification implies that a neurological disease has not been ruled out, or that one has been identified but that the disability is out of proportion to it. That this label is applied to schizophrenia seems inappropriate, given that there is no conclusive evidence that it is a neurological disease.

5   McNally, *A Critical History of Schizophrenia*, 2016, pp. 5–6.

6   McNally, *A Critical History of Schizophrenia*, 2016, p. 5.

7   E.g. N. Coulon, O. Godin, E. Bulzacka, C. Dubertret, J. Mallet, G. Fond, L. Brunel, M. Andrianarisoa, G. Anderson, I. Chereau, H. Denizot, R. Rey, J. M. Dorey, C. Lançon, C. Faget, P. Roux, C. Passerieux, J. Dubreucq, S. Leignier, D. Capdevielle, M. André, B. Aouizerate, D. Misdrahi, F. Berna, P. Vidailhet, M. Leboyer, F. Schürhoff, 'Early and very early-onset schizophrenia compared with adult-onset schizophrenia: French FACE-SZ database', *Brain Behav.* 10(2) (2020). doi: 10.1002/brb3.1495.

8   Ibid.

9   J. Moncrieff, H. Middleton, 'Schizophrenia: a critical psychiatry

perspective', *Current Opinion Psychiatry*. 28(3) (2015), pp. 264–8. doi: 10.1097/YCO.0000000000000151.

10 APA, 1980, 6.

11 Kępińska, Adrianna P et al. 'Schizophrenia polygenic risk predicts general cognitive deficit but not cognitive decline in healthy older adults', *Translational psychiatry* vol. 10,1 422 (2020) doi:10.1038/s41398-020-01114-8

12 W. C. Corning & R. A. Steffy, 'Taximetric strategies applied to psychiatric classification', *Schizophrenia Bulletin*, 5(2) (1979), pp. 294–305. doi.org/10.1093/schbul/5.2.294 quoted in McNally, 2016, p. 206.

13 J. T. Braslow, J. S. Brekke, J. Levenson, 'Psychiatry's myopia-reclaiming the social, cultural, and psychological in the psychiatric gaze', *JAMA Psychiatry* 78 (4) (2021) p. 349. doi.org/10.1001/jamapsychiatry.2020.2722; Dumas-Mallet, E., Gonon, F., 'Messaging in biological psychiatry: misrepresentations, their causes, and potential consequences', *Harv. Rev. Psychiatry* 28 (6) (2020), pp. 395–403; C. Gardner, A. Kleinman, 'Medicine and the mind – the consequences of psychiatry's identity crisis', *N. Engl. J. Med.* 381 (18) (2019), pp. 1697–1699; Scull, A., 'American psychiatry in the new millennium: a critical appraisal', *Psychol. Med.* (2021), pp. 1–9.

14 N. Andreason, *The Broken Brain*, 1984.

15 Quoted in Harrington, 2019, p. xiii

16 J. Van Os '"Schizophrenia" does not exist', *BMJ* 352 (2016):i375 doi:10.1136/bmj.i375.

17 Jay Joseph, *Schizophrenia and Genetics: The End of An Illusion* (London: Routledge, 2023).

18 J. Moncrieff, H. Middleton, 'Schizophrenia: a critical psychiatry perspective', *Curr Opin Psychiatry*. 28(3) (2015), pp. 264–8. doi: 10.1097/YCO.0000000000000151.

19 Richard Bentall and David Pilgrim, There are no 'schizophrenia genes': here's why', *The Conversation* (April 8, 2016).

20 E. Fuller Torrey, 'Did the Human Genome Project Affect Research on Schizophrenia?' *Psychiatry Research* (2023) doi.org/10.1016/j.psychres.2023.115691.

21 T. Fall, R. Kuja-Halkola, K. Dobney, et al. 'Evidence of large genetic influences on dog ownership in the Swedish Twin Registry has implications for understanding domestication and health associations', *Sci Rep* 9, 7554 (2019). doi.org/10.1038/s41598-019-44083-9; Chia-chen Chang, Thi Phuong Le Nghiem, Qiao Fan,

Notes

Claudia L. Y. Tan, Rachel Rui Ying Oh, Brenda B. Lin, Danielle F. Shanahan, Richard A. Fuller, Kevin J. Gaston, L. Roman Carrasco, 'Genetic Contribution to Concern for Nature and Proenvironmental Behavior', *BioScience*, Volume 72, Issue 2 (2022), pp. 160–165, doi.org/10.1093/biosci/biab103

22 M. Farrell, T. Werge, P. Sklar, P, et al. 'Evaluating historical candidate genes for schizophrenia', *Mol Psychiatry* 20 (2015), pp. 555–562. doi. org/10.1038/mp.2015.16; E. C. Johnson et al., 'No Evidence That Schizophrenia Candidate Genes Are More Associated With Schizophrenia Than Noncandidate Genes', 82, 10 (2017), pp. 702–708, doi.org/10.1016/j.biopsych.2017.06.033; P F Sullivan, 'How Good Were Candidate Gene Guesses in Schizophrenia Genetics?' *Biological Psychiatry*, Volume 82, Issue 10 (2017), pp. 696–697. doi. org/10.1016/j.biopsych.2017.09.004

23 Marsman A, Pries LK, ten Have M, de Graaf R, van Dorsselaer S, Bak M & van Os J. 'Do current measures of polygenic risk for mental disorders contribute to population variance in mental health?' *Schizophrenia Bulletin*, sbaa086 (2020) doi.org/10.1093/schbul/sbaa086

24 A. Rammos, L. A. N. Gonzalez, D. R. Weinberger, K. J. Mitchell & K. K. Nicodemus, 'The role of polygenic risk score gene-set analysis in the context of the omnigenic model of schizophrenia', *Neuropsychopharmacology* (2019). doi:10.1038/s41386-019- 0410-z in www.madinamerica.com/2020/08/genetics-may-predict-o-5-schizophrenia/

25 A. Sekar, A. R. Bialas, H. de Rivera, A. Davis, T. R. Hammond, N. Kamitaki, K. Tooley, J. Presumey, M. Baum, V. Van Doren, G. Genovese, S. A. Rose, R. E. Handsaker, 'Schizophrenia Working Group of the Psychiatric Genomics Consortium'; M. J. Daly, M. C. Carroll, B. Stevens, S. A. McCarroll, 'Schizophrenia risk from complex variation of complement component 4', *Nature* 530(7589) (2016), pp. 177–83. doi: 10.1038/nature16549. Epub 2016 Jan 27. Erratum in: *Nature* 601(7892) (2022):E4-E5.

26 Noel Hunter, 'Breaking News! The Cause of Schizophrenia Finally Discovered!(?)' *Mad in America* (3 February 2016).

27 Rajiv Radhakrishnan, Muzaffer Kaser, Sinan Guloksuz, 'The Link Between the Immune System, Environment, and Psychosis', *Schizophrenia Bulletin*, Volume 43, Issue 4 (2017), pp. 693–697. doi. org/10.1093/schbul/sbx057; N. Muller, A. M. Myint, M. J. Schwarz,

'Inflammation in schizophrenia', *Advances in Protein Chemistry and Structural Biology*, 88 (2012). pp. 49–68.

28 P. S. Bloomfield, S. Selvaraj, M. Veronese, G. Rizzo, A. Bertoldo, D. R. Owen & O. D. Howes, 'Microglial activity in people at ultra high risk of psychosis and in schizophrenia: An [11C]PBR28 PET brain imaging study', *The American Journal of Psychiatry*, 173(1) (2015), pp. 44–52.

29 O. S. Kowalczyk et al, 'Neurocognitive correlates of working memory and emotional processing in postpartum psychosis: an fMRI study', *Psychological Medicine* 51 (2021), pp. 1724–1732. doi. org/10.1017/ S0033291720000471.

30 Katie Hazelgrove, Alessandra Biaggi, Freddie Waites, Montserrat Fuste, Sarah Osborne, Susan Conroy, Louise M. Howard, Mitul A. Mehta, Maddalena Miele, Naghmeh Nikkheslat, Gertrude Seneviratne, Patricia A. Zunszain, Susan Pawlby, Carmine M. Pariante, Paola Dazzan, 'Risk factors for postpartum relapse in women at risk of postpartum psychosis: The role of psychosocial stress and the biological stress system', *Psychoneuroendocrinology*, Volume 128 (2021), 105218,ISSN 0306-4530, doi.org/10.1016/j. psyneuen.2021.105218; M. Aas, C. Vecchio, A. Pauls, M. Mehta, S. Williams, K. Hazelgrove, A. Biaggi, S. Pawlby, S. Conroy, G. Seneviratne, V. Mondelli, C. M. Pariante, P. Dazzan, 'Biological stress response in women at risk of postpartum psychosis: The role of life events and inflammation', *Psychoneuroendocrinology* 113:104558 (2020). doi: 10.1016/j.psyneuen.2019.104558.

31 A. Danese, C. M. Pariante, A. Caspi, A. Taylor, R. Poulton, 'Childhood maltreatment predicts adult inflammation in a life-course study', *Proc Natl Acad Sci U S A* 104(4) (2007), pp. 1319–24. doi: 10.1073/pnas.0610362104.

32 S. R. Dube, D. Fairweather, W. S. Pearson, V. J. Felitti, R. F. Anda & J. B. Croft, 'Cumulative childhood stress and autoimmune diseases in adults', *Psychosomatic Medicine*, 71(2) (2009), pp. 243–250.

33 C. Heim, U. M. Nater, E. Maloney, R. Boneva, J. F. Jones & W. C. Reeves, 'Childhood trauma and risk for chronic fatigue syndrome', *Archives of General Psychiatry*, 66(1) (2009), pp. 72–80.

34 John Read and Pete Sanders, *A Straight Talking Introduction To The Causes Of Mental Health Problems* (2nd Edition) (Monmouth, PCCS Books, 2010); E.g. Filippo Varese, Feikje Smeets, Marjan Drukker, Ritsaert Lieverse, Tineke Lataster, Wolfgang Viechtbauer, John Read, Jim van Os, Richard P. Bentall, 'Childhood Adversities

Increase the Risk of Psychosis: A Meta-analysis of Patient-Control, Prospective- and Cross-sectional Cohort Studies', *Schizophrenia Bulletin*, Volume 38, Issue 4 (2012), pp. 661–671: doi.org/10.1093/schbul/sbs050, Jay Joseph, 'The Schizophrenia Genetics Illusion – A Century of Failure and Hype', *Mad in America* (12 December 2022).

35 O. Ajnakina, A. Trotta, E. Oakley-Hannibal, M. Di Forti, S. A. Stilo, A. Kolliakou & C. Pariante, 'Impact of childhood adversities on specific symptom dimensions in first-episode psychosis', *Psychological Medicine*, 46(2) (2016), pp. 317–326.

36 I. Janssen, L. Krabbendam, M. Bak, M. Hanssen, W. Vollebergh, R. de Graaf & J. van Os, 'Childhood abuse as a risk factor for psychotic experiences', *Acta Psychiatrica Scandinavica*, 109 (2004), pp. 38–45.

37 R. Bentall, S. Wickham, M. Shevlin & F. Varese, 'Do specific early-life adversities lead to specific symptoms of psychosis? A study', *Schizophrenia Bulletin*, 38 (2012), pp. 734–740 cited in Noel Hunter, 'Breaking News! The Cause of Schizophrenia Finally Discovered!(?)' *Mad in America* (3 February 2016).

38 Ibid.

39 C. Morgan, G. Knowles, G. Hutchinson, 'Migration, ethnicity and psychoses: evidence, models and future directions', *World Psychiatry* 18(3) (2019), pp. 247–258.

40 A. Tortelli, A. Errazuriz, T. Croudace, et al. 'Schizophrenia and other psychotic disorders in Caribbean-born migrants and their descendants in England: systematic review and meta-analysis of incidence rates, 1950–2013', *Soc Psychiatry Psychiatr Epidemiol;*50 (2015), pp. 1039–55.

41 J. P. Selten, N. Veen, W. Feller et al. 'Incidence of psychotic disorders in immigrant groups to The Netherlands', *Br J Psychiatry* 178 (2001), pp. 367–72; Veling W, Selten JP, Veen N et al. 'Incidence of schizophrenia among ethnic minorities in the Netherlands: a four-year first-contact study', *Schizophr Res* 86 (2006), pp. 189–93.

42 Wim Veling, Jean-Paul Selten, Ezra Susser, Winfried Laan, Johan P Mackenbach, Hans W Hoek, 'Discrimination and the incidence of psychotic disorders among ethnic minorities in The Netherlands', *International Journal of Epidemiology*, Volume 36, Issue 4 (2007), pp. 761–768.

43 J. P. Selten, W. Laan, R. Kupka et al. Erratum to: 'Risk of psychiatric treatment for mood disorders and psychotic disorders among migrants and Dutch nationals in Utrecht, The Netherlands', *Soc*

Psychiatry Psychiatr Epidemiol 50, 167–169 (2015): doi.org/10.1007/s00127-014-0964-3.

44 J. B. Kirkbride, D. Barker, F. Cowden et al. 'Psychoses, ethnicity and socio- economic status', *Br J Psychiatry* 193 (2008), pp. 18–24.

45 A. C. Hollander, H. Dal, G. Lewis et al. 'Refugee migration and risk of schizophrenia and other non-affective psychoses: cohort study of 1.3 million people in Sweden', *BMJ* 352 (2016):i1030.

46 F. Termorshuizen, E. van der Ven, I. Tarricone et al. 'The incidence of psychotic disorder among migrants and ethnic minority groups in Europe: findings from the multinational EU-GEI study', *Psychol Med.* 52(7) (2022), pp. 1376–1385: doi: 10.1017/S0033291720003219.

47 P. Fearon, J. B. Kirkbride, C. Morgan et al. 'Incidence of schizophrenia and other psychoses in ethnic minority groups: results from the MRC AESOP Study', *Psychological Medicine.* 36(11) (2006), pp. 1541–1550: doi:10.1017/S0033291706008774.

48 Morgan et al. *World Psychiatry*, 2019, pp. 247–258.

49 J. McGrath, S. Saha, J. Welham et al. 'A systematic review of the incidence of schizophrenia: the distribution of rates and the influence of sex, urbanicity, migrant status and methodology', *BMC Med* 2:13 (2004). Cantor-E. Graae, J. P. Selten, 'Schizophrenia and migration: a meta-analysis and review', *Am J Psychiatr* 162 (2005), pp. 12–24; F. Bourque, E. van der Ven, A. Malla, 'A meta-analysis of the risk for psychotic disorders among first- and second-generation immigrants', *Psychol Med* 41 (2011), pp. 897–910; M. C. Castillejos, C. Martin-Perez, B. Moreno-Kustner, 'A systematic review and meta-analysis of the incidence of psychotic disorders: the distribution of rates and the influence of gender, urbanicity, immigration and socio-economic level', *Psychol Med* (in press); H. E. Jongsma, C. Turner, J. B. Kirkbride et al. 'International incidence of psychotic disorders, 2002–17: a systematic review and meta-analysis', *Lancet Public Health* 2019;4:e229-44; J. P. Selten, E. van der Ven, F. Termorshuizen, 'Migration and psychosis: a meta-analysis of incidence studies', *Psychol Med* (in press); E. van der Ven, W. Veling, A. Tortelli et al. 'Evidence of an excessive gender gap in the risk of psychotic disorder among North African immigrants in Europe: a systematic review and meta-analysis', *Soc Psychiatry Psychiatr Epidemiol* 51 (2016), pp. 1603–13; A. Tortelli, A. Errazuriz, T. Croudace et al. 'Schizophrenia and other psychotic disorders in Caribbean-born migrants and their descendants in England: systematic review and meta-analysis of incidence rates, 1950–2013',

Soc Psychiatry Psychiatr Epidemiol 50 (2015), pp. 1039–55; J. B. Kirkbride, A. Errazuriz, J. T. Croudace et al. 'Incidence of schizophrenia and other psychoses in England, 1950–2009: a systematic review and meta-analyses', *PLoS One* 2012;7:e31660.

50 Matthew Lewin, 'Schizophrenia "epidemic" among African Caribbeans spurs prevention policy change', *Guardian* (9 December 2009).

51 J. M. Eagles, 'The relationship between schizophrenia and immigration. Are there alternatives to psychosocial hypotheses?' *Br J Psychiatry* 159 (1991), pp. 783–9.

52 Morgan et al, 2019.

53 R. J. Barrett, 'Conceptual foundations of schizophrenia: I. Degeneration', *Australian and New Zealand Journal of Psychiatry* 32 (1998), pp. 617–26.

54 Ibid.

55 S. Mahone and M. Vaughan (eds), *Psychiatry and Empire* (Basingstoke: Palgrave Macmillan UK, 2007) in *Mad World*, 2023, p. 58.

56 Metzl, *The Protest Psychosis.*, Ibid.

57 American Psychiatric Association, *DSM-ii: Diagnostic and Statistical Manual of Mental Disorders*, second edition (1968).

58 P. Fearon, J. Kirkbride, C. Morgan, et al. 'Incidence of schizophrenia and other psychoses in ethnic minority groups: results from the MRC ÆSOP Study', *Psychol Med*, 36:11 (2006), pp. 1541–50.

59 Elizabeth Cantor-Graae, Ph.D., and Jean-Paul Selten, Ph.D., M.D, 'Schizophrenia and Migration: A Meta-Analysis and Review', *American Journal of Psychiatry*, Volume 162, Number 1 (2005): doi: org/10.1176/appi.ajp.162.1.12.

60 J. van Os, S. Guloksuz, 'A critique of the "ultra-high risk" and "transition" paradigm', *World Psychiatry* 16(2) (2017), pp. 200–206. doi: 10.1002/wps.20423; van Os J, Kenis G, Rutten BP. 'The environment and schizophrenia', *Nature* 468(7321) (2010), pp. 203–12. doi: 10.1038/nature09563.

61 J. van Os, U. Reininghaus, 'Psychosis as a transdiagnostic and extended phenotype in the general population', *World Psychiatry* 15(2) (2016), pp. 118–24. doi: 10.1002/wps.20310.

62 Guloksuz S, Pries LK, Ten Have M, de Graaf R, van Dorsselaer S, Klingenberg B, Bak M, Lin BD, van Eijk KR, Delespaul P, van Amelsvoort T, Luykx JJ, Rutten BPF, van Os J. 'Association of preceding psychosis risk states and non-psychotic mental disorders

with incidence of clinical psychosis in the general population: a prospective study in the NEMESIS-2 cohort', *World Psychiatry*, 19(2) (2020), pp. 199–205. doi: 10.1002/wps.20755.

63 Van Os, www.chapeau-woonkringen.nl/documenten/artikelen/150307_NRC_Jim_van_Os.pdf

64 Ibid

65 J. van Os, P. Galdos, G. Lewis, M. Bourgeois, A. Mann, 'Schizophrenia sans frontieres: concepts of schizophrenia among French and British psychiatrists', *BMJ*, 307(6902) (1993), pp. 489–92. doi: 10.1136/bmj.307.6902.489.

66 http://www.chapeau-woonkringen.nl/documenten/artikelen/150307_NRC_Jim_van_Os.pdf

67 L. Phahladira, H. K. Luckhoff, L. Asmal et al. 'Early recovery in the first 24 months of treatment in first-episode schizophrenia-spectrum disorders', *NPJ Schizophr* 6, 2 (2020). doi.org/10.1038/s41537-019-0091-y.

68 S. Kapur, A. G. Phillips, T. R. Insel, 'Why has it taken so long for biological psychiatry to develop clinical tests and what to do about it?' *Mol. Psychiatry*, 17 (12) (2012), pp. 1174–1179 in Jim van Os, Sinan Guloksuz, 'Schizophrenia as a symptom of psychiatry's reluctance to enter the moral era of medicine', *Schizophrenia Research*, Volume 242 (2022), pp. 138–140. doi.org/10.1016/j.schres.2021.12.017.

69 J. van Os, A. C. J. Kohne, 'It is not enough to sing its praises: the very foundations of precision psychiatry may be scientifically unsound and require examination', *Psychological Medicine*, 51(9) (2021), pp. 1415–1417. doi: 10.1017/S0033291721000167.

70 www.schizofreniebestaatniet.nl/english/; www.psychosenet.nl

71 About Hearing Voices Network: www.hearing-voices.org/about-us/

72 One example is neuroleptic malignant syndrome (NMS), characterised by sweating, fever, tremors, difficulty speaking and swallowing, a rapid heart rate, and changes in consciousness, including confusion and lethargy, stupor or coma.

73 Steven Hyman quoted in Harrington, 2019, p. xv.

74 Harrington, 2019, p. xiv.

7: New Frontiers: Psychedelics

1 'Tim Ferriss, the Man who put his Money behind Psychedelic Medicine', *The New York Times*, (September 2019).

2 'Psychedelic medicine', *Nature* (28 September 2022).

Notes

3   'Tim Ferriss, the Man who put his Money behind Psychedelic
    Medicine', *The New York Times*, (September 2019).

4   Elias A. Zerhouni, 'Translational and Clinical Science: Time for a
    New Vision', *New England Journal of Medicine*, 2005, p. 1622, in
    Robinson, 2019, p. 3.

5   For a history, see Pollan, Michael, *This Is Your Mind on Plants
    (London: Penguin, 2021)*.

6   J. Phelps, R. N. Shah & J. A. Lieberman, 'The rapid rise in
    investment in psychedelics – Cart before the horse. *JAMA
    Psychiatry*, 79(3) (2022), pp. 189–190. doi.org/10.1001/
    jamapsychiatry.2021.3972.

7   E.g. J. S. Aday, B. D. Heifets, S. D. Pratscher, E. Bradley, R. Rosen & J.
    D. Woolley, 'Great Expectations: Recommendations for improving
    the methodological rigor of psychedelic clinical trials',
    Psychopharmacology, 239(6) (2022), p. 1989–2010: doi.org/10.1007/
    s00213-022-06123-7; M. Butler, L. Jelen & J. Rucker, 'Expectancy in
    placebo-controlled trials of psychedelics: If so, so what?'
    Psychopharmacology, 239(10) (2022), pp. 3047–3055: doi.org/10.1007/
    s00213-022-06221-6; S. D. Muthukumaraswamy, A. Forsyth & T.
    Lumley, 'Blinding and expectancy confounds in psychedelic
    randomized controlled trials', *Expert Review of Clinical
    Pharmacology*, 14(9) (2021), pp. 1133–1152: doi.org/10.1080/17512433.20
    21.1933434, cited in J. Davies, B. A. Pace & N. Devenot, 'Beyond the
    psychedelic hype: Exploring the persistence of the neoliberal
    paradigm', *Journal of Psychedelic Studies* (2023): doi.
    org/10.1556/2054.2023.00273.

8   D. Nutt, D. Erritzoe & R. Carhart-Harris, 'Psychedelic psychiatry's
    brave new world', *Cell*, 181(1) (2020), pp. 24–28: doi.org/10.1016/j.
    cell.2020.03.020.

9   J. Davies, B. A. Pace & N. Devenot, 'Beyond the psychedelic hype:
    Exploring the persistence of the neoliberal paradigm', *Journal of
    Psychedelic Studies* (2023): doi.org/10.1556/2054.2023.00273.

10 Clay Skipper, 'From Productivity to Psychedelics: Tim Ferriss Has
    Changed His Mind About Success', *GQ* (22 July 2020).

11 Clay Skipper, 'From Productivity to Psychedelics: Tim Ferriss Has
    Changed His Mind About Success', *GQ* (22 July 2020).

12 Huxley qtd. in Steven J. Novak, 'LSD Before Leary: Sidney Cohen's
    Critique of 1950s Psychedelic Drug Research', *Isis* 88, no. 1 (1977):
    95, in Harrington, 2019, p. 151.

13 Olivia Goldhill, 'It's a "psychedelic renaissance," as scientists identify medicinal qualities of hardcore drugs', GQ (May 22, 2016).

14 Peter Grinspoon, MD, 'Back to the future: Psychedelic drugs in psychiatry', *Harvard Health Publishing* (22 June 2021); Ronit Molko, 'Psychedelics As Treatment Options For Mental Health', *Forbes* (19 May 2022); Laura Newberry, 'The 'gnarly and painful' therapeutic potential of 'magic mushrooms', *Los Angeles Times* (14 February 2023).

15 Harrington, 2019, p. 152

16 American Women Since 1954, 1987, Rochelle Gatlin, p. 97

17 R. L. Carhart-Harris et al. 'Psilocybin with psychological support for treatment-resistant depression: an open-label feasibility study', *Lancet Psychiatry* 3 (2016), pp. 619–627; R. L. Carhart-Harris et al. 'Psilocybin with psychological support for treatment-resistant depression: six-month follow-up', *Psychopharmacology* 235 (2018), pp. 399–408; L. Roseman, D. J. Nutt & R. L. Carhart-Harris, 'Quality of acute psychedelic experience predicts therapeutic efficacy of psilocybin for treatment-resistant depression', *Front. Pharmacol.* 8, 974 (2017); O. G. Bosch, S. Halm & E. Seifritz, 'Psychedelics in the treatment of unipolar and bipolar depression', *Int J Bipolar Disord* 10, 18 (2022): doi.org/10.1186/s40345-022-00265-5.

18 R. R. Griffiths et al. 'Psilocybin produces substantial and sustained decreases in depression and anxiety in patients with life-threatening cancer: a randomized double-blind trial', *J. Psychopharmacol.* 30 (2016), pp. 1181–1197; J. D. McCorvy, R. H. Olsen & B. L. Roth, 'Psilocybin for depression and anxiety associated with life-threatening illnesses', *J. Psychopharmacol.* 30 (2016), pp. 1209–1210.

19 G. Jones, J. A. Ricard, J. Lipson et al. 'Associations between classic psychedelics and opioid use disorder in a nationally-representative U.S. adult sample', *Sci Rep* 12, 4099 (2022): doi.org/10.1038/s41598-022-08085-4; M. W. Johnson, A. Garcia-Romeu, R. R. Griffiths, 'Long-term follow-up of psilocybin-facilitated smoking cessation', *Am J Drug Alcohol Abuse*, 43(1) (2017), pp. 55–60: doi: 10.3109/00952990.2016.1170135. Erratum in: *Am J Drug Alcohol Abuse*, 43(1) (2017), p. 127; M. P. Bogenschutz, A. A. Forcehimes, J. A. Pommy, C. E. Wilcox, P. Barbosa, R. J. Strassman, 'Psilocybin-assisted treatment for alcohol dependence: A proof-of-concept study', *Journal of Psychopharmacology*, 29(3) (2015), pp. 289–299: doi:10.1177/0269881114565144; Garcia-A. Romeu, A. K. Davis, E.

Erowid, F. Erowid, R. R. Griffiths and M. W. Johnson, 'Persisting Reductions in Cannabis, Opioid, and Stimulant Misuse After Naturalistic Psychedelic Use: An Online Survey', *Front. Psychiatry* 10:955. (2020): doi: 10.3389/fpsyt.2019.00955.

20 J. Halifax, *Shamanic voices: A survey of visionary narratives. Wondrous medicine* (New York: Penguin, 1979) pp. 125–135) in J. R. George, T. I. Michaels, J. Sevelius & M. T. Williams, 'The psychedelic renaissance and the limitations of a White-dominant medical framework: A call for indigenous and ethnic minority inclusion', *Journal of Psychedelic Studies*, 4(1) (2020), pp. 4–15. doi: org/10.1556/2054.2019.015.

21 J. W. Allen, *María Sabina: Saint Mother of the Sacred Mushrooms* (Ethnomycological Journals, vol. 1) (Seattle, WA: Psilly Publications, 1997).

22 R. G. Wasson, *The Wondrous Mushroom: Mycolatry in Mesoamerica* (San Francisco, CA: City Light Publishers, 2014).

23 I use the term 'indigenous', echoing the work of George, Michaels, Sevelius and Williams cited, to refer specifically to members of ethnic groups who are original settlers of or native to a particular country or region, as opposed to more recently settled groups who may have colonised the area. The indigenous use of psychedelics, these authors also note, cannot be mapped on to modern geographic and national boundaries. Its history should be considered as tied to a broader community of indigenous practices across North, Central and South Americas that were ultimately appropriated primarily by Western clinicians and scientists.

24 Clay Skipper, 'From Productivity to Psychedelics: Tim Ferriss Has Changed His Mind About Success', GQ (22 July 2020).

25 N. Chwelos, D. B. Blewett, C. M. Smith et al. Use of d-lysergic acid diethylamide in the treatment of alcoholism', *Q J Stud Alcohol* 20 (1959), pp. 577–90; R. Yensen, F. B. Di Leo, J. C. Rhead et al. 'MDA-assisted psychotherapy with neurotic outpatients: A pilot study', *J Nerv Ment Dis* 163 (1976), pp. 233–45; K. W. Tupper, E. Wood, R. Yensen, M. W. Johnson, 'Psychedelic medicine: a re-emerging therapeutic paradigm', *CMAJ* 6;187(14) (2015), pp. 1054–1059: doi: 10.1503/cmaj.141124; Vittoria D'Alessio, 'Psychedelics paired with therapy could treat chronic mental health conditions', *Horizon* (24 October 2022).

26 Shayla Love, 'Investors Are Debating Who Should Own the Future of Psychedelics', *Vice* (10 March 2021).

27 M. Leamy, V. Bird, C. Le Boutillier et al. 'Conceptual framework for personal recovery in mental health: systematic review and narrative synthesis', *Br J Psychiatry* 199 (2011), pp. 445–52; S. R. Stuart, L. Tansey, E. Quayle, 'What we talk about when we talk about re- covery: a systematic review and best-fit framework synthesis of qualitative literature', *J Ment Health* 26 (2017), pp. 291–304;Van Os, Jim et al., 'The evidence-based group-level symptom-reduction model as the organizing principle for mental health care: time for change?' *World Psychiatry*;18 (2019) 88–96.

28 K. A. MacLean, M. W. Johnson & R. R. Griffiths, 'Mystical experiences occasioned by the hallucinogen psilocybin lead to increases in the personality domain of openness', *Journal of Psychopharmacology*, 25(11), (2011), pp. 1453–1461: doi. org/10.1177/0269881111420188; D. Erritzoe, V. G. Frokjaer, K. K. Holst, M. Christoffersen, S. S. Johansen, C. Svarer & G. M. Knudsen, 'Serotonergic psychedelics LSD & psilocybin increase the personality trait of openness', *Journal of Psychopharmacology*, 34(9) (2020), pp. 989–999: doi.org/10.1177/0269881120908005; R. R. Griffiths, W. A. Richards, U. McCann & R. Jesse, 'Psilocybin can occasion mystical-type experiences having substantial and sustained personal meaning and spiritual significance', *Psychopharmacology*, 187(3) (2006), pp. 268–283. doi.org/10.1007/s00213-006-0457-5; E. Studerus, M. Kometer, F. Hasler & F. X. Vollenweider, 'Acute, subacute and long-term subjective effects of psilocybin in healthy humans: a pooled analysis of experimental studies', *Journal of Psychopharmacology*, 25(11) (2011), pp. 1434–1452. doi.org/10.1177/0269881110382466.

29 S. Ross, et al., 'Rapid and sustained symptom reduction following psilocybin treatment for anxiety and depression in patients with life-threatening cancer: a randomized controlled trial', *Journal of Psychomarmacology*, 30 (12) (2016), pp. 1165–1180.

30 B. E. Wampold, 'How important are the common factors in psychotherapy? An update', *World Psychiatry* 14 (2015), pp. 270–7; B. R. Rutherford, M. M. Wall, A. Glass et al. 'The role of patient expectancy in placebo and nocebo effects in antidepressant trials', *J Clin Psychiatry* 75 (2014), pp. 1040–6; S. Kam-Hansen, M. Jakubowski, J. M. Kelley et al. 'Altered placebo and drug labelling changes the outcome of episodic migraine attacks', *Sci Transl Med* 6:218ra5 (2014); S. A. Baldwin, Z. E. Imel, 'Therapist effects: findings and methods' in: Lambert MJ (ed). *Bergin and Garfield's Handbook*

of Psychotherapy and Behavior Change, 6th ed. (New York: Wiley, 2013), pp. 258–97; Jim Van Os et al., 'The evidence-based group-level symptom-reduction model as the organizing principle for mental health care: time for change?' *World Psychiatry* 18 (2019), pp. 88–96.

31 J. J. Breeksema, B. W. Kuin, J. Kamphuis, W. van den Brink, E. Vermetten, R. A. Schoevers, 'Adverse events in clinical treatments with serotonergic psychedelics and MDMA: A mixed-methods systematic review', *J Psychopharmacol* 36(10) (2022), pp. 1100–1117. doi: 10.1177/02698811221116926.

32 Jim Van Os et al., 'The evidence-based group-level symptom-reduction model as the organizing principle for mental health care: time for change?' *World Psychiatry*, 18 (2019), pp. 88–96.

33 Dan Baum, 'Legalize It All: How to win the war on drugs', *Harper's Magazine* (April 2016).

34 Pollan, *This Is Your Mind on Plants*, *(London: Penguin Books, 2021)*

35 Dan Baum, 'Legalize It All: How to win the war on drugs', *Harper's Magazine* (April 2016).

36 D. Merica, 'Trump declares opioid epidemic a national public health emergency', *CNN* (26 October 2017). Retrieved from www.cnn.com/2017/10/26/politics/donald-trump-opioid-epidemic/index.html

37 J. Netherland & H. Hansen, 'White opioids: Pharmaceutical race and the war on drugs that wasn't. *Biosocieties*, 12(2) (2017), pp. 217–238: doi:10.1057/biosoc.2015.46.

38 J. J. Palamar, S. Davies, D. C. Ompad, C. M. Cleland & M. Weitzman, 'Powder cocaine and crack use in the United States: An examination of risk for arrest and socioeconomic disparities in use', *Drug and Alcohol Dependence*, 149 (2015), pp. 108–116: doi:10.1016/j.drugalcdep.2015.01.029 in J. R. George, T. I. Michaels, J. Sevelius & M. T. Williams, 'The psychedelic renaissance and the limitations of a White-dominant medical framework: A call for indigenous and ethnic minority inclusion', *Journal of Psychedelic Studies*, 4(1) (2020), pp. 4–15. doi: org/10.1556/2054.2019.015

39 Owen Bowcott and Frances Perraudin, 'BAME offenders "far more likely than others" to be jailed for drug offences', *Guardian* (15 January 2020).

40 M. Alexander, *The New Jim Crow: Mass Incarceration in the Age of Colorblindness* (New York: New Press, 2010) in J. R. George, T. I Michaels, J. Sevelius & M. T Williams, 'The psychedelic renaissance

and the limitations of a White-dominant medical framework: A call for indigenous and ethnic minority inclusion', *Journal of Psychedelic Studies*, 4(1) (2020), pp. 4–15: doi. org/10.1556/2054.2019.015

41   J. Forman, 'Racial critiques of mass incarceration: Beyond the new Jim Crow', *New York University Law Review*, 87(1) (2012), pp. 101–146. Retrieved from www.digitalcommons.law.yale.edu/cgi/ viewcontent.cgi?article=4599=fss_papers

42   D. H. Suite, R. La Bril, A. Primm & P. Harrison-Ross, 'Beyond misdiagnosis, misunderstanding and mistrust: Relevance of the historical perspective in the medical and mental health treatment of people of color'. *Journal of the National Medical Association*, 99(8) (2007), pp. 879–878.

43   A. M. Brandt, 'Racism and research: The case of the Tuskegee syphilis study', *Hastings Center Report*, 8(6) (1978), pp. 21–29: doi:10.2307/3561468; V. S. Freimuth, S. C. Quinn, S. B. Thomas, G. Cole, E. Zook & T. Duncan, 'African Americans' views on research and the Tuskegee Syphilis study', *Social Science and Medicine*, 52(5) (2001), pp. 787–808: doi:10.1016/S0277-9536(00)00178-7.

44   M. T. Williams & C. Leins, 'Race-based trauma: The challenge and promise of MDMA-assisted psychotherapy', *Multidisciplinary Association for Psychedelic Studies (MAPS) Bulletin*, 26(1) (2016), pp. 32–27.

45   M. T. Williams, D. Printz, T. Ching & C. T. Wetterneck, 'Assessing PTSD in ethnic and racial minorities: Trauma and racial trauma', *Directions in Psychiatry*, 38(3) (2018), pp. 179–196.

46   T. I. Michaels, J. Purdon, A. Collins & M. T. Williams, 'Inclusion of people of color in psychedelic-assisted psychotherapy: A review of the literature', *BMC Psychiatry*, 18(245) (2018), pp. 1–9: doi:10.1186/ s12888-018-1824-6.

47   Shayla Love, 'Investors Are Debating Who Should Own the Future of Psychedelics', *Vice* (10 March 2021).

48   J. R. George, T. I. Michaels, J. Sevelius & M. T. Williams, 'The psychedelic renaissance and the limitations of a White-dominant medical framework: A call for indigenous and ethnic minority inclusion', *Journal of Psychedelic Studies*, 4(1) (2020), pp. 4–15: doi. org/10.1556/2054.2019.015.

49   Leia Friedwoman, 'Male Supremacy and the Psychedelic Patriarchy', *The Psychedologist* (16 May 2018).

50 G. Herzberg & J. Butler, 'Blinded by the White: Addressing power and privilege in psychedelic medicine', *Chacruna* (2019).

8: Neurodiversity as a Model for Care

1   At most, 10 per cent of autistic people have so-called savant abilities, although about half of savants are autistic. See: Darold A. Treffert, 'The savant syndrome: an extraordinary condition. A synopsis: past, present, future', *Philosophical transactions of the Royal Society of London. Series B, Biological sciences* vol. 364,1522 (2009), pp. 1351–7: doi:10.1098/rstb.2008.0326.

2   I use 'woman' here for people who identify as women, and so are likely to experience the social demands particular to upholding a female gender identity in a Western social context.

3   R. McCrossin, 'Finding the True Number of Females with Autistic Spectrum Disorder by Estimating the Biases in Initial Recognition and Clinical Diagnosis', *Children (Basel)*, 9(2) (2022), p. 272: doi: 10.3390/children9020272.

4   American Psychiatric Association. *Diagnostic and Statistical Manual of Mental Disorders (DSM-5)*. (Washington, DC: American Psychiatric Association Publishing, 2013).

5   Amelia Hill, '"Diagnosis is rebirth": women who found out they were autistic as adults', *Guardian* (19 November 2021).

6   Hannah Devlin, '"We weren't visible": Growing awareness leads more women to autism diagnosis', *Guardian* (19 Nov 2021).

7   G. Russell, S. Stapley, T. Newlove-Delgado, A. Salmon, R. White, F. Warren, A. Pearson and T. Ford, 'Time trends in autism diagnosis over 20 years: a UK population-based cohort study', *J Child Psychol Psychiatr*, 63 (2022), pp. 674–682: doi.org/10.1111/jcpp.13505.

8   'More Girls are Being Diagnosed with Autism', *The New York Times* (14 Apr 2023).

9   M. C. Lai, S. Baron-Cohen & J. D. Buxbaum, 'Understanding autism in the light of sex/gender', *Molecular Autism* 6, 24 (2015): doi. org/10.1186/s13229-015-0021-4.

10 S. Jacquemont, B. P. Coe, M. Hersch, M. H. Duyzend, N. Krumm, S. Bergmann, J. S. Beckmann, J. A. Rosenfeld, E. E. Eichler, 'A higher mutational burden in females supports a 'female protective model' in neurodevelopmental disorders', *Am J Hum Genet*, 94(3) (2014), pp. 415–25: doi: 10.1016/j.ajhg.2014.02.001.

11 'NIH awards $100 million for Autism Centers of Excellence Program', *National Institutes of Health* (4 September 2012)

12 E.g Apoorva Mandavilli, 'The Invisible Women with Autism', *The Atlantic* (22 October 2015).

13 Ibid.

14 E.g. H. Wood-Downie, B. Wong, H. Kovshoff et al. 'Sex/Gender Differences in Camouflaging in Children and Adolescents with Autism', *J Autism Dev Disord* 51 (2021), pp. 1353–1364: doi. org/10.1007/s10803-020-04615-z; J. Gould, 'Towards understanding the under-recognition of girls and women on the autism spectrum. *Autism*, 21(6) (2017), pp. 703–705: doi.org/10.1177/1362361317706174; P. Corscadden & A. M. Casserly, 'Identification of Autism in Girls: Role of Trait Subtleties, Social Acceptance and Masking. *REACH: Journal of Inclusive Education in Ireland*, 34(1) (2021).

15 M. Dean, R. Harwood & C. Kasari, 'The art of camouflage: Gender differences in the social behaviors of girls and boys with autism spectrum disorder', *Autism*, 21(6) (2017), pp. 678–689: doi. org/10.1177/1362361316671845; C. Tomlinson, C. Bond & J. Hebron, 'The mainstream school experiences of adolescent autistic girls', *European Journal of Special Needs Education*, 37(2) (2022), pp. 323–339: doi.org/10.1080/08856257.2021.1878657.

16 A. Rynkiewicz, I. Łucka, 'Autism spectrum disorder (ASD) in girls. Co-occurring psychopathology. Sex differences in clinical manifestation', *Psychiatr. Pol.* 52(4) (2018), pp. 629–639; Caitlin Murray, Hanna Kovshoff, Anthony Brown, Patricia Abbott, Julie A. Hadwin, 'Exploring the anxiety and depression profile in individuals diagnosed with an autism spectrum disorder in adulthood', *Research in Autism Spectrum Disorders*, Volume 58, (2019), pp. 1–8, ISSN 1750-9467: doi.org/10.1016/j.rasd.2018.11.002.

17 Hansman-Wijnands MA, Hummelen JW. 'Differentiële diagnostiek van psychopathie en autismespectrumstoornissen bij volwassenen [Differential diagnosis of psychopathy and autism spectrum disorders in adults. Empathic deficit as a core symptom]', *Tijdschr Psychiatr.* 48(8) (2006), pp. 627–36. Dutch. PMID: 16958304.

18 E.g. Hannah Devlin, '"We weren't visible": Growing awareness leads more women to autism diagnosis', *Guardian* (19 Nov 2021); 'More Girls are Being Diagnosed with Autism', *The New York Times* (14 Apr 2023).

19 Apoorva Mandavilli, 'The Invisible Women with Autism', *The Atlantic* (22 October 2015).

20 E.g. Siobhan Tierney, Jan Burns, Elizabeth Kilbey, 'Looking behind the mask: Social coping strategies of girls on the autistic spectrum,

Research in Autism Spectrum Disorders', Volume 23 (2016), pp. 73–83.

21 M. Dekker, 'On our own terms: Emerging autistic culture,' *Conference paper*, Aitism99 (1999).

22 Mitzi Waltz, *Autism: A Social and Medical History*, (Springer, 2013), p. 136.

23 Ibid.

24 M. Dekker, 'On our own terms: Emerging autistic culture,' *Conference paper*, Aitism99 (1999).

25 Ibid.

26 *Our Voice*, Volume 1, Number 3, 1993.

27 E.g. Autism Speaks, 'Autism & Your Family.' New York: Autism Speaks, 2012. Online at: www.autismspeaks.org/what-autism/autism-your-family.

28 *Our Voice*, Volume 1, Number 3, 1993.

29 Mitzi Waltz, *Autism: A Social and Medical History*, 2013, p. 136.

30 J. E. Robison, 'My Time with Autism Speaks' in: S. Kapp, (eds) *Autistic Community and the Neurodiversity Movement* (Singapore: Palgrave Macmillan, 2020).

31 Mitzi Waltz, *Autism: A Social and Medical History*, 2013, p. 138.

32 'Horrific Autism Speaks "I am Autism" ad transcript', *ASAN* (23 September 2009).

33 Sulivan (pseudonym of M. J. Carey) 'Autism Research Funding: Who's Paying and How Much?' *Left Brain Right Brain: Autism News Science and Opinion* (21 July 2009). Online at: http://leftbrainrishtbrain.co.uk/2009/07/autism. research-funding-who-is-paying-and-how-much, in Waltz, 2013, p. 138.

34 Autism Speaks has been blocked in the UK – its former UK branch is now known as Autistica, and has a very different agenda to its parent charity (and an autistic director).

35 Sulivan (pseudonym of M. J. Carey) 'Autism Research Funding: Who's Paying and How Much?' *Left Brain Right Brain: Autism News Science and Opinion* (21 July 2009). Online at: http://leftbrainrishtbrain.co.uk/2009/07/autism. research-funding-who-is-paying-and-how-much, in Waltz, 2013, p. 138.

36 ABA is the only autism intervention that is approved by insurers and Medicaid in all fifty states. ABA often targets autistic traits that are harmless, such as fidgeting and avoiding eye contact, because they are perceived to be socially stigmatising. Children are rewarded for 'good' behaviour, often with treats. While some

parents, in particular, find the approach beneficial in helping their children acquire skills like communicating, and waiting, many autistic people find the treatment dehumanising. ABA can help autistic people manage environments with neurotypical people, but the dominance of this approach prevents discussions about how these environments can better accommodate autistic people, nor does it address the issues that are most urgent to autistic people themselves, to help them thrive, and not merely fit in. In a conformist society, individuals or their parents might turn to ABA to prevent more violent forms of constraint, sectioning or police intervention. This makes it necessary for many in order to survive the reality of a broken social system, but it doesn't mean that we do not need better options and real support that goes beyond teaching people to mask or suppress their experience, wherever they fall on the spectrum. For a discussion of ABA, see: www.newyorker.com/ science/annals-of-medicine/ the-argument-over-a-long-standing-autism-intervention

37 Harrington, 2019, p. 179.
38 M. Dawson. 'Seminar: In conversation with Michelle Dawson,' London: Centre for Research and in Autism and Education, Institute of Education, University of London, 2012.
39 S. M. Robertson, 'Neurodiversity, quality of life, and autistic adults:
40 Shifting research and professional focuses onto real-life challenges,' *Disability Studies Quarterly*, 30 (1) (2010).
41 Ibid.
42 Sally Ozonoff, PhD, Gregory S. Young, PhD, Alice Carter, PhD, Daniel Messinger, PhD, Nurit Yirmiya, PhD et al, 'Recurrence Risk for Autism Spectrum Disorders: A Baby Siblings Research Consortium Study', *Pediatrics* 128 (3) (2011) e488–e495: doi. org/10.1542/peds.2010-2825
43 Marta Zaraska, 'The problems with prenatal testing for autism', *The Transmitter* (14 August 2019).
44 Wei-Ju Chen et al. 'Autism Spectrum Disorders: Prenatal Genetic Testing and Abortion Decision-Making among Taiwanese Mothers of Affected Children', *International journal of environmental research and public health* vol. 17,2 476. (2020): doi:10.3390/ijerph17020476; 'A routine prenatal ultrasound can identify early signs of autism, study finds', Science Daily (9 February 2022); Schwarz, E., Guest, P., Rahmoune, H. et al. 'Sex-specific serum biomarker patterns in

adults with Asperger's syndrome', *Mol Psychiatry* 16 (2011), pp. 1213–1220: doi.org/10.1038/mp.2010.102.

45 'Unprecedented Academic-Industry Collaboration Seeks New Drugs and Novel Treatments for Autism,' *Autism Speaks* (19 March 2012). Online at: http://www.autismspeaks.org/about-us/press-releases/ research-academic-industry-drugs-discovery.

46 Chrystiane V.A. Toscano, Leonardo Barros, Ahlan B. Lima, Thiago Nunes, Humberto M. Carvalho, Joana M. Gaspar, 'Neuroinflammation in autism spectrum disorders: Exercise as a "pharmacological" tool', *Neuroscience & Biobehavioral Reviews*, Volume 129 (2021) pp. 63–74, ISSN 0149-7634: doi.org/10.1016/j.neubiorev.2021.07.023; Eissa, Nermin et al. 'Role of Neuroinflammation in Autism Spectrum Disorder and the Emergence of Brain Histaminergic System. Lessons Also for BPSD?' *Frontiers in pharmacology* vol. 11 886. (2020): doi:10.3389/fphar.2020.00886; Matta SM, Hill-Yardin EL, Crack PJ. 'The influence of neuroinflammation in Autism Spectrum Disorder', *Brain Behav Immun* 79 (2019), pp. 75–90: doi: 10.1016/j.bbi.2019.04.037.

47 David Cox, 'Are we ready for a prenatal screening test for autism?' *Guardian* (1 May 2014).

48 Heide Aungst, 'New Research Shows How Brain Inflammation in Children May Cause Neurological Disorders Such as Autism or Schizophrenia', *University of Maryland School of Medicine* (12 October 2023).

49 See: Chess S. 'Autism in children with congenital rubella', *J Autism Child Schizophr.* 1971 Jan-Mar;1(1) (1971), pp. 33–47: doi: 10.1007/BF01537741 and follow-up report: Chess S. 'Follow-up report on autism in congenital rubella', *J Autism Child Schizophr.* 7(1) (1977), pp. 69–81: doi: 10.1007/BF01531116.

50 'Factsheet about congenital rubella syndrome', *European Centre for Disease Prevention and Control* (2023): www.ecdc.europa.eu/en/congenital-rubella-syndrome/facts

51 F. Marques, M. J. Brito, M. Conde, M. Pinto, A. Moreira, 'Autism spectrum disorder secondary to enterovirus encephalitis', *J Child Neurol.* 29(5) (2014), pp. 708–14: doi: 10.1177/0883073813508314.

52 See: Stephen Barrett, M.D., 'The Rise and Fall of CARE Clinics and the Center for Autistic Spectrum Disorders (CASD)', *Autism Watch* (6 February 2018).

53 Barrett S. 'Commercial hair analysis. Science or scam?' *JAMA*. 30;254(8) (1985), pp. 1041–5.
54 https://swanscotland.org/about-us

Conclusion: The Other Side
1 Sanah Ahsan, 'I'm a psychologist – and I believe we've been told devastating lies about mental health' *Guardian* (6 Sep 2022).
2 Rose, 2019, p. 146
3 D. Bhugra, A. Tasman, S. Pathare, S. Priebe, S. Smith, J. Torous, M. R. Arbuckle, A. Langford, R. D. Alarcón, and H. F. K. Chiu, 'The WPA-Lancet Psychiatry Commission on the Future of Psychiatry', *The Lancet Psychiatry*, 4(10) (2017), pp. 775–818.; Rose, 2019.
4 Rose, 2019, p. 192.
5 Bhugra et al., 2017; Rose, 2019, p. 177.
6 Rose, 2019, p. 180.
7 Rose, 2019, p. 196

Acknowledgements

This book was a challenge to write, because it meant a lot to me that it did justice to the perspectives and experiences it encompasses.

From the beginning, I could rely on the support of my agent, Eli Keren, and my editor at Profile, Izzy Everington, in shaping what felt like an ambitious contribution to the debates on mental health. I am so grateful for Izzy's edits and support as the book took shape, and also to Zara Sehr Ashraf at Profile for her thoughtful insights.

Most of all, though, my thinking on mental health has evolved through the conversations with the people affected by, and involved in, psychiatry. I have so much appreciation for the people quoted in this book, who have had encounters with psychiatric treatment, and who have bravely and kindly shared their stories with me. Their visions of a more caring mental healthcare system, their expertise and initiatives, form the hopeful backbone to this book. My thanks also to the psychiatrists and other mental healthcare professionals who have spoken on the areas and the people they have dedicated their lives to, as well as their candid statements on the challenges of their work.

So much has changed in my own life since I first wrote the proposal for this book. My family and friends have been a constant, and I'm so happy I have them. Luong has been a new addition, and I couldn't have imagined what a support he would be. I hope they can all see the love they have shown me reflected in these pages.

Index

LSD and mescaline 197–8
magic mushrooms 200–201
origin story 200–201
peer support and 205–6
personalised treatment 210
potential of 194–5
psilocybin 200–202, 208–9
psychedelic renaissance 197, 213
reciprocal relationships and
204–5
recovery narratives aided by
psychedelic retreats 207–8
researchers exaggerate positive
results and hide risks 195
set and setting and 202–3
Shroom Boom 196
term 196–7
therapy, proven only in
combination with 202
'woah, man' statements 196
psychiatry
access to support 4, 78, 88, 97,
140, 152, 158, 162, 189, 199,
204–5, 213, 214, 216, 245, 249,
251
anti-psychiatry movement 43,
94–5
big pharma and 47–8, 49–52
biomedical model for mental
health/medical view of
mental suffering see
biomedical model
black people and see black
people and black women
'cult-like' status of 3
Diagnostic and Statistical
Manual of Mental Disorders
(DSM) and see Diagnostic
and Statistical Manual of
Mental Disorders (DSM)

drugs/medications and see
individual drugs/medication
name
minority groups and see
minority groups
neuroscience and see
neuroscience
origins of 11–40, 160
social determinants of mental
health and see social
determinants of mental
health
women and see women
See also individual condition
name
psychoanalysis 21–2, 44, 85, 185,
237
psychopathy 8, 74, 76, 121–54, 225,
253
antisocial personality disorder
(ASPD) and 130, 132, 133, 134,
140
arrogant and deceitful
interpersonal style and 125
bisexual men or women and
132
black people and 129–30, 132,
139–40
borderline personality disorder
and 130, 138–9, 143
children and adolescents 141–2,
144–9
Chromis and 142, 153
communities, impact on 137,
138, 139, 140, 141, 142, 143, 144,
145, 146, 148, 150, 152, 153, 154
Comprehensive Assessment of
Psychopathic Personality
(CAPP) 134–7
culture and symptoms of 125–6